Pranayama

Breathing Techniques to Kundalini Awakening

(Master the Art of Pranayama Breathing and the Ujjayi Breath)

Peter Beamon

Published By **Phil Dawson**

Peter Beamon

Pranayama: Breathing Techniques to Kundalini Awakening (Master the Art of Pranayama Breathing and the Ujjayi Breath)

ISBN 978-1-77485-807-3

Legal & Disclaimer

Table Of Contents

Chapter 1: Yoga - What is Yoga?

Yoga comes from the Sanskrit word "yug", which literally means to bind.

It is a holistic way to live that unites our body, mind, soul and spirit to make us happier, more balanced, and more harmonious. This union can lead to a communion of individual consciousness and the universal power/universal reality.

According to Yogic scriptures Shiva, a Hindu deity, was the first Yogi who achieved the state of supreme awareness. The knowledge was passed on to his seven disciples, known as Sapta Rishis. They were seven Sages who spread the knowledge through word of mouth in ancient India.

Patanjali (another great sage) was the first person to collect and codify yoga in 196 Yoga Sutras, or aphorisms, in and around 200 B.C. These 196 Sutras are divided in four chapters: - Samadhi Pad, Sadhan pad and Vibhutipad, Kaivalyapad. This provides a framework that allows for spiritual growth as well as mastery over the mental and physical bodies.

Patanjali stated that yoga's primary objective is to slow down the mind to allow transformation and attain the highest level of consciousness, called samadhi. These yoga sutras have become the basis of modern yoga.

Later, many other gurus or teachers contributed to preservation and development of yoga. There were various schools of yoga that embraced and tied religion to yoga practice, such as Bhakti Yoga, Mantra Yoga, and Mantra Yoga.

Chapter 2: Types of Yoga

Many schools of yoga are based on how they approach yoga and what they do to achieve the ultimate goal. Some examples are:

1. Karma Yoga

2. Bhakti Yoga

3. Hatha Yoga

4. Kundalini Yoga

5. Mantra Yoga

6. Dhyana Yoga

7. Jain Yoga

8. Bodh Yoga

9. Patanjal Yoga

Meditation (dhyana), or concentration, is a common form of yoga. It can be used to attain enlightenment. There are many different meditation focus options. Meditation on one or more chakras such as the heart center (anahata), third eye (ajna), and meditation based in religion are all possible. However, the end goal remains unchanged: attaining the highest degree of enlightenment.

Chapter 3: Ashtanga Yoga

Patanjal yoga does not have any religious or religious affiliations, even though it is certain that yoga originated in Hindu tradition.

Patanjali, a great sage or maharishi, composed the eight fold path from his book Patanjal Yoga Sutras. In his second sutra, he defined the goal and definition of yoga as follows:

"chitta vritti nirodha"

This is also known as "the cessation mental fluctuations".

Ashtanaga Yoga is the most popular and closely followed descendent to Patanjal. It is also known as rajyoga. Ashtanga's origins are two Sanskrit phrases, "Ashta + Anga".

"Ashta," which means eight, is pronounced "Anga," which means limbs. It can also be translated as Eight Limb Path.

Eight Limbs Ashtanga Yoga

1. Yama – Principles or moral code

i. Ahimsa means nonviolence in thought or action. Anxiety is a violent emotion.

ii. Satya - Truthfulness in thoughts and speech.

iii. Asteya is prohibited from stealing.

iv. Brahmcharya: Celibacy, regulating sexual indulgence.

v. Aparigraha

2. Niyama - Disciplines.

Saucha: Cleanliness and purity in all aspects, inner and external-physical and psychological.

ii. Santosh, Contentment, To Be at Peace

iii. Tapa: Endurance

iv. Swadhaya: Self-study, self-reflection

v. Eshwar Pranidhan: Dedication

3. Asana is a series of postures or positions that help you to stay mentally and physically stable.

This is the most common aspect of yoga. Asanas have many benefits including improved flexibility, strength and balance. The deeper benefits of asana are that it calms the mind and prepares the ground for spiritual experiences.

4. Pranayama – Regulation of breath, Controlling Breath.

Yoga Sutras teaches that pranayama, asana, and other practices can be used to purify the mind and increase self-discipline.

5. Pratyahara-Withdrawal of the senses.

Pratyahara in yoga refers to the letting go or releasing the senses from attachments to external objects or sources. This is the way to self-realization, inner peace and tranquility.

6. Dharana - Concentration.

It is the act to focus or center our attention on a single object (third eye chakra tip of nose or any mental image).

This state is reached when one has completely disconnected the minds and physical senses – pratyahara. After withdrawal, you can focus your mind and energy on the object rather than being distracted by the physical senses.

7. Dhayana - Meditation.

We have all seen it happen. The mind can become focused, but the mind has a tendency to wander after a while.

Dharana can be described as concentration. Dhayana, on the other hand, is continuous concentration which makes our inner consciousness more powerful.

8. Samadhi = Self-realization of Salvation or Moksha

This is the highest state in inner consciousness that produces a state known as trance. It is a state when mind becomes one.

Things to remember before you try yoga

1. Yoga can be done at any time during the day. Yoga is most effective when done in the morning. You can make a difference in your health by doing daily yoga in morning.

2. Practice asanas when you have nothing to eat.

3. It is important to practice in a calm, quiet environment that allows you to relax your body and mind.

4. You can practice asanas with a relaxed mindset, paying attention to your body and breath. No jerky movements.

5. Do not hold your poses for too long if you are just starting out. Listen to your body, and let go of any asanas that cause pain or discomfort.

6. Yoga does not only include stretching. Yoga can also include relaxation, meditation, breathing, mindfulness, and other aspects.

7. Breathe through your nose, and after you have reached a steady place, bring awareness to your breathing and body.

8. Before beginning yoga, your doctor should be consulted if you are suffering from any chronic condition or ailment.

9. You can reap the full benefits of yoga by doing it every day for 15-30 minutes, instead of 3 sessions for 1hr each week.

Relaxation with Mudras, Pranayamas and Asanas

Yoga is holistic and works on all facets of the person. It can be a powerful cognitive booster that can not only reduce stress or anxiety but also help you live a balanced and harmonious life.

Yoga practice begins with breath awareness. Deeper, more conscious breaths calm the mind, draw attention inward and allow us to become more aware our inner thoughts, desires, experiences, and feelings.

For the best results, your yoga practice should incorporate the following three. :-

1. Mudras are hand positions.

2. Pranayama, or breath awareness, is an example of Pranayama.

3. Asana (yoga poses)

Combining all three practices together can bring calmness and balance to every level of our being, including the emotional and mental. It can also be used to balance and energize the chakras that contain energy.

For beginners, you can begin by practicing each one and then incorporate them into your daily practice as you feel more comfortable.

Let's learn about mudras pranayama, asanas, and more.

Chapter 4: Mudras

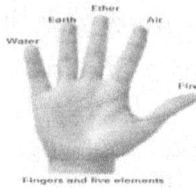

Fingers and five elements

In Sanskrit, mudra means "gesture" or "attitude".

Yogis used mudras to activate chakras and energy centers in their bodies. Mudras aid in energy flow by clearing blockages. Both mental and bodily ailments can be caused when there is a blockage. If energy flows freely, our bodies feel great.

The five types of yoga mudras are broadly divided into the following:

1. Hasta, or the Hand mudras

2. Mana or head mudras

3. Kaya and Postural mudras

4. Bandha or Lock mudras

5. Adhara or Perineal mudras

We will be focusing mainly upon hasta Mudras.

Hasta Mudras (hand gestures or positions) are used for energy balance. They can redirect energy back to the body, restore health, and help to balance out energy. According to yogic philosophy our body is made up of five elements, earth, water and fire as well as air and ether. Our fingers represent each element.

The thumb is made of fire (manipura/solarplexus chakra), the index fingers are air (anahata/heart Chakra), the middle finger ether (vishuddha/thorugh chakra) and the ring is earth (muldhara, the root chakra). While the little finger is water ("swadhisthana")

Every finger that comes in contact with the thumb will bring balance to the affected element. This can help heal the disease. To reap the benefits, it is recommended that you hold the positions for 30 minutes. However, if you are just starting to exercise your fingers, any time will do.

Mudras, which are simple gestures that can enhance meditation, are powerful. These positions are very easy to integrate into your daily activities. You can do them anywhere and anytime you like, including standing, walking, traveling, watching your favorite shows, and even sitting down. The next 21 days, you should aim to practice at least 30 minutes of mudras each day.

Let's review some basic mudras that we can incorporate into our daily yoga practice, to enhance our meditation experience and to energize our chakras.

Gyan Mudra, Mudra of Knowledge

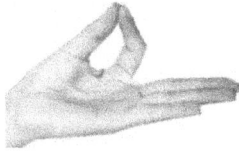

This powerful mudra involves touching the tip the index finger with your thumb. Relax the rest of your fingers. This mudra increases your body's air element. You can do it anywhere and anytime. It is most commonly used for meditation, or to perform some asanas such Vajrasana, Sukhasana.

Benefits:-

This mudra, which has been used by yogis for thousands upon thousands of years, enhances meditation and concentration. It helps to reduce negativity and promote peace, calm spiritual growth, spiritual growth, sharpening memory, and stimulating the root chakra.

Akash Mudra, Mudra of Space

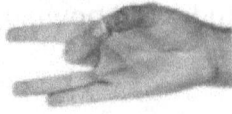

This detoxifying mudra involves touching the tip your middle finger with the tip you thumb. Relax the three other fingers. This mudra increases your body's ether (or space) element.

Benefits:-

This mudra is good for developing intuition and increased sensory power. It stimulates the throat chakra and purifies thoughts and emotions. It helps to eliminate metabolic wastes from the body and relieves congestion caused by migraines.

Prithvi Mudra – Mudras for Earth

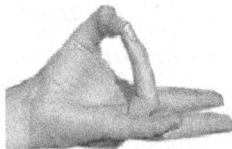

This mudra can be created by touching the tip the ring finger with your thumb. Relax the three other fingers. This mudra can used anywhere, anytime.

16

Benefits:-

It improves energy and decreases tiredness. It improves patience, self-assurance, stability, and perseverance.

Yoni Mudra – Mudra Of Womb Or Source

This mudra is created by interlocking your middle, little and ring finger. Place your thumbs together, and point them away form the body. Connect the thumbs of the index fingers and point them downwards towards the base of a "yoni" or womb shape.

Benefits:-

This mudra increases stability in meditation by stabilizing the mind and body. It helps increase concentration, awareness, as well as balancing the activities between the left and right brain hemispheres. It not only creates balance but also redirects energy away from the body through the fingers and hands.

Chapter 5: Pranayama

"When the breathing wanders, the mind also becomes unsteady." But when the mind is calmed, it will be steady." Svatmarama HathaYoga Pradipika

"Prana" stands for the vital energy or universal force of life, or the breath. 'Ayama' is the term used to control or regulate.

Pranayama means control of your breath, or the art of breathing. Pranayama is mainly done through your nose. There are three steps to pranayama.

1. Inhalation of Poraka

2. Retention (kumbhaka).

3. Exhalation

Pranayama (or fourth limb) is a part of ashtanagayoga. Patanjali in his Yoga Sutras text mentioned pranayama among the essential means of reaching higher states of awareness.

Pranayama helps us to do our asanas well. Blockage of prana (or energy) is commonly attributed to stiffening the body in yogic cultures. This can lead to toxicity accumulation. The toxins can be flushed out of the system by prana or energy flowing through them. This improves flexibility and overall health.

Let us now learn about some pranayama techniques that can rejuvenate our bodies and respiratory systems.

Bhramari Pranayama - Humming Bee Breath

Bhramari, a variety Indian honey bee, is one example.

This is a relaxing pranayama, which takes its name form the Bhramari bee. This pranayama is reminiscent of the sound of a honeybee when it's exhaled.

How to practice pranayama

a. Sit straight in a calm, peaceful, and comfortable location.

b. Cover your eyes completely with all your fingers. Block your ears with the thumbs.

c. Take a deep breath in. Breathe in deeply and make a buzzing sound like a bee. This can be achieved by simply chanting "om", without speaking.

d. Keep inhaling and keep going for around 5 to 10 more times.

Benefits:-

It is a great way to calm your mind. It increases memory and concentration.

Anulom Valom – Alternate Breathing

Anulom Vilom means 'alternate' or' reversed'.

This pranayama balances the breathing by only using one nostril. This allows the other nostril to be closed by closing it with your fingers. The thumb and the middle finger are used for closing the nostril.

How to practice pranayama

a. Place yourself in a tranquil, quiet, and comfortable position.

b. Keep your right thumb close to the right nostril and inhale air from the left nostril. Keep going until your lungs are full.

c. Next, release the thumb with your right hand. Breathe slowly through the right nostril.

d. Next, exhale air through the right nostril.

After closing the right nostril and touching the left ring-finger, inhale through the left nostril.

F. This refers to one round of Anulom Vilom Pranayama. Start with four rounds. You can increase this number by adding more rounds to make it 10 rounds in a single session.

Start slow and keep the inhalation/exhalation rhythm to 4 counts. Once you feel confident, then increase the time between exhalation (inhalation) and exhalation to 2 seconds.

Benefits:-

It helps release anxiety and stress by calmening the mind. Right nostril breathing activates our sympathetic nervous systems, and left activates our parasympathetic system. This alternate breathing allows for a balance of both the parasympathetic and sympathetic nervous systems.

Kapalbhati Pranayama - Shining forehead

Kapal refers to the forehead and bhati refers to shining or glowing.

This activating pranayama is where deep inhalation is followed by forceful expiration. This cleanses the body of toxins and purifies blood. This makes your skin look beautiful and healthy.

How to practice pranayama

a. In a calm, quiet and comfortable environment, stand straight.

b. You should ensure that your spine is straight.

c. Your hand can be placed on your belly.

d. Breathe deeply and feel the air rise in your stomach.

E. Slowly pull your stomach inwards as you exhale. You should pull your navel towards your spine like you are pushing the air out.

f. Repeat the circuit 5-10 times.

Benefits:-

The pranayama cleanses the lungs and revitalizes the cells. This is a good exercise for toning the stomach. Pranayama, especially for ladies, rejuvenates your cells. This helps reduce wrinkles and gives you a glowing and healthy complexion.

Asanas

In Sanskrit, asana means "posture" or "position".

Asanas can also be practiced sitting, standing, kneeling, and lying down. They are mainly performed while standing, sitting, or kneeling. They should be slow, steady, and not jerky.

A posture involves three main stages:

1. Get into the right posture

2. Staying in the position

3. You can return to your original position.

Asanas should always be done with awareness of the body and breath. The body should have a coordinated movement between breath and movements. Inhale as you raise any part and exhale as you lower your body. Asanas can be held for as long or as little as you feel comfortable, depending on your personal limitations. Do not force yourself to do more than you can.

Patanjali's Yoga Sutras defines yoga asanas as

"Sthiram sukham aasanam"

This results in a more comfortable, relaxing, and steady position.

You should not expect to master the pose within the first day. Find the pose that works best for you. Don't let yourself be judged. Do not try to achieve perfection in the first day. For beginners, you should start with the easiest asanas. You should listen to your body and choose a position that is comfortable and natural for you. When practicing your poses, be calm and keep your breathing steady. You should master at least one of your poses before you can move onto the next.

Asanas Lying on Stomach: Back Asanas

Shavasana - Corpse Pose

In Sanskrit, Shava means Corpse.

This position allows for complete relaxation and rest.

These are the steps to practicing asana

a. Start by lying down on your back on the mat.

b. Close your eyes.

c. Bend your arms at a 45° angle. Alternatively, place your hands on the palms of your hands or in Gyan Mudra/Prithvi

Mudra. Allow the feet to relax towards the sides.

d. Make your head aligned with your spine.

e. Let go of all worries and focus on the breath. Take a deep, slow breath. Now pay attention to your body.

f. Now, relax by paying attention to each organ in your body from head and toe.

Be free from any fears, worries, or conflicts that you may have by focusing only on yourself, and not the world around.

Benefits: -

This poses calms the mind and reduces stress and fatigue. It is also good for reducing anxiety, blood pressure and insomnia. The third eye, or "ajna chakra", is the best place to focus in order to energize the chakra. This pose is great for after work or before bed. Alternate with Advasana (Reverse Corpse position) or Jyestikasana.

Setu Bandha Sarvangasana - Bridge Pose

In Sanskrit, setu means bridge; bandha means energy-binder.

This pose refers to an energy bridge.

These are the steps to practicing asana

a. Start by lying down on your back on the mat.

b. Be sure to keep your arms apart from the body.

c. Bend at the knees and bring in your heels as far as you can towards your hips.

d. Spread your arms out with your palms facing upwards.

e. Exhale, and press down on the ground with your feet. Next, lift your lower back up, middle back, and upper back off to the floor. Keep your spine parallel to ground.

f. Concentrate on your breathing and continue to breathe easily. You can hold this position for up to eight breaths. Then, release slowly.

g. Take a deep breath and relax into the pose.

To support your lower back, place a block of your hands or your hands below it.

Benefits: -

This pose calms your brain and helps reduce stress, anxiety, and depression. It stimulates your thyroid and digestion. It also strengthens back muscles and gives good stretch to the spine, neck, and chest. Physically, it's a great exercise to tone your stomach muscles and help you energize the "vishuddha", the fifth chakra.

Viparita Karani - Legs Up Pose

In Sanskrit, viparita means "inverted" or "reversed"; karani means "doing" or "making".

This pose is easy for beginners. You can support yourself with a wall. You won't need support from the wall once you feel comfortable and improve your practice.

These are the steps to practicing asana

a. As a beginner, place your left hand against a wall.

b. Slowly lean backward, then swing your legs towards the wall.

c. Inhale, and then adjust the position of the tailbone so that it is as close as possible to the wall.

d. Close you eyes and focus on your breath.

e. You can hold this pose for about a minute.

f. Let go of this position by gently rolling on your side.

With practice, you will be able to perform this pose without any support from the wall.

Benefits: -

This pose is good for overall health and well-being. It calms the nervous system and strengthens the immune system. This helps to balance the hormonal system, stabilize the digestion and eliminate system, and it also energizes the "ajna", which is the sixth chakra (the third eye).

Makarasana - Crocodile Pose

In Sanskrit, Makar means crocodile.

This pose looks a lot like crocodiles lying on their stomachs with their heads slightly elevated.

These are the steps to practicing asana

a. Lie on your stomach and chest.

b. Spread the legs at full length.

c. Elevate the head and chest. Bend your elbows to extend the arms and rest your elbows on the ground.

d. Create a cup shape by using both of your hands. Place the head on your heels.

e. Close you eyes and breathe deeply.

f. Aim to relax the body and bring awareness to your lower back.

Benefits: -

This pose is good for relaxation, especially in the lower back. This pose helps to activate the "manipura", a third chakra that is located close to the navel.

Bhujangasana - Cobra Pose

Bhujang means Snake or cobra in Sanskrit.

This pose is so named because the raised head and neck look like a cobra lifting its hood.

These are the steps to practicing asana

a. Lay on your stomach, with your forehead towards the ground. Your arms should be extended forward to your side.

b. As you inhale, raise your arms towards your chest. You don't have to lift your waist as a beginner. Do some practice to get comfortable with the position.

c. Keep your elbows straight, if you can. Beginners might need to bend their elbows slightly. Avoid putting too much pressure on your hands. Hands and arms should only be used for balance and support.

d. Relax and breathe deeply. Keep your buttocks from clenching.

e. Take a deep breath and exhale.

Start slowly by holding the pose for five second. When you are more comfortable, gradually increase the time.

Benefits: -

This pose increases flexibility and strengthens the spine. The thyroid gland can be stimulated by stretching the head and neck back. It opens your chest to facilitate inhalations. It is also known to help tone the abdomen, buttocks, as well as helping to energize the "Swadhisthana", or the second chakra.

Sitting Asanas

Sukhasana: Easy Sitting Pose

Sukh refers to joy, happiness.

This is the best position to sit for beginners. It is an excellent asana for meditation or deep breathing. In this pose, Gyan Mudra can also be used.

These are the steps to practicing asana

a. Place your legs straight in front and sit on the mat. If you need extra support, you might place a pillow under your hips.

b. Fold the left foot and place it under the right leg.

c. Now fold the right knee and place it under the left.

d. Keep straight spine.

e. Keep both hands on the knees.

You are welcome to incorporate a mudra or pranayama with this pose.

f. Close all eyes and relax.

Practice this pose for at minimum 5 minutes, focusing on your breathing.

Benefits: -

This poses strengthens the back and stretch the knees, ankles, and hips. It can help calm your mind and reduce stress. You can achieve Padamasana with regular practice.

Vajrasana - Thunderbolt pose

In Sanskrit, Vajra means thunder bolt.

It is a meditative position.

These are the steps to practicing asana

a. Place your feet on your heels, and fold your legs.

b. Be sure to keep your hips up with the heels.

c. Keep the thighs covered

d. Make certain your spine is straight.

e. Keep your hands on the hips.

f. Pay attention and focus on your breathing.

Benefits: -

This pose can calm the mind, aid in digestion, and help combat constipation. This pose is the main one for Anandmadirasana (or Bliss Pose) and Ardh Utstrasana (or Camel Pose).

Shishuasana -- Child Pose

Shishu refers to a child.

This relaxing pose is a great one for relaxation.

These are the steps to practicing asana

a. Place your heels on a mat.

b. Keep your hips on heels. Now, bend forward and lower you forehead towards the mat.

c. Keep your hands together by your side, palms facing out or in Gyan Modra

d. Close you eyes and gently press down on your thighs.

e. Keep your attention on your breath. Listen to the sound of your inhale, exhale, and focus on your breath.

f. Slowly lift your heels up and sit down on the heels.

Benefits: -

This pose increases your physical, emotional and mental vitality. It increases blood circulation to the head and calms your body and nervous system. It can also open the hips and stretch the lower back.

Ardha Matsyendrasana - Half Spinal Twist

Ardha is half, Matsyendra the king.

This is a seated spine twist asana.

These are the steps to practicing asana

a. Start in Sukhasana.

b. Bend the left leg, and place your heel beside your right hip.

c. Lift your right leg up above your left knee. The right foot's toes should face forward.

d. Put your left hand on your right knee, and your right hand behind.

e. Breathe deeply and turn your waist, shoulders, and neck slowly to right. Then look over the right side shoulder.

f. Maintain a straight spine.

g. Breathe freely and consciously.

h. Take a deep breath and then let it out.

You can start by doing it on each side. Then, gradually increase your holding time to one minute for each side.

Benefits: -

This pose opens your chest and increases oxygen flow to the body. It is also a great way to detoxify, relax the mind and revitalize your body. It increases the elasticity in the spine, and it stretches and contracts the muscles of one side and the abdomen on the other.

Paschimottanasana - Forward Bend

Paschim means "west"; ottana mean "stretch".

This posture can be used to reduce stress by relaxing the spine muscles and helping to calm the mind.

These are the steps to practicing asana

a. Sit straight up, with your spine straightening and your toes pointed upwards.

b. Relax your body. Exhale, raise your hands above your head, and stretch.

c. Breathe in and lower your arms. Bend forward to touch your feet. Do not move forward in abrupt or jerky ways.

d. You can grasp your toes with your fingers if you're able. If this does not feel right, you can always place your fingers wherever it is most comfortable. As far forward as you feel comfortable. Forward bending is an important asana that stretches the back muscles. It does not stretch the head on the knees.

Breathe in, and lengthen your spine. As you exhale, hold your navel near your knees.

During this asana you should keep your back muscles loose.

f. Keep your attention on your breath, lower back, abdomen and chest.

g. To get started, hold the pose for 5 second to determine if it is comfortable. If not, increase the holding time.

Slowly return to the beginning position.

Start with two rounds of this pose as a beginner.

Benefits: -

This pose helps calm the brain and reduces stress and mild depression. It reduces fatigue and anxiety as well as relieving headaches and anxiety. It strengthens the spine and shoulders as well as the hamstrings. It stimulates the entire abdomen including the liver, pancreas and adrenal glands.

Standing Asanas

Tadasana - Mountain Pose

Tad means mountain.

This pose represents the stability and might of a mountain. It is also a great pose to use for Utkatasana or other asanas.

These are the steps to practicing asana

a. Standing with your feet slightly apart, get up and stand.

b. Use your fingers to interlock and then raise them as one unit slowly.

c. If you don't want to lock your fingers at first, you can simply raise your hand.

d. Elevate your heels from the floor and balance on your feet.

e. While you are in this position, hold it for 5-10 seconds and breathe deeply.

Although it can be hard to maintain balance at the start, it will become easier with practice.

f. Exhale, bring the heels to the ground and release interlocking fingers.

Benefits: -

This pose is good for bringing stability to the body. It also improves balance, self awareness, and breathing. This pose offers a vertical stretch to all your body muscles. It helps in energizing the "Muldhara", which is the root chakra. This brings about inner peace, security, and calm.

Utkatasana -- Chair Pose

Utkat refers to intense or powerful.

This is a difficult pose that resembles sitting on an imaginary seat.

These are the steps to practicing asana

a. Place your feet slightly apart while standing straight.

b. Stretch your arms out, but don't bend your elbow.

c. Breathe in and extend your legs, pushing your pelvis forward as if you're sitting on a chair.

d. Keep both your hands parallel to ground and straighten your back.

e. Bend slowly but not so fast that your knees reach your toes.

f. Inhale deeply and consciously.

Benefits: -

The pose is good for building willpower, and it has an energizing impact on both body and mind. It strengthens your lower back and tone your legs and thighs while burning fat. It helps to activate the "muldhara", the root chakra.

Vrikshasana, Tree Pose

In Sanskrit, Vriksh means tree.

This pose is similar to a tree. A tree can move with wind and it's okay to start off a little unsteady before you reach a balance.

These are the steps to practicing asana

a. Get up on your mat in a standing position.

b. Keep your eyes on the front.

c. Hold your hands on your hips while inhaling deeply.

d. Place your right leg up high, and then place it on your left thigh.

e. After you feel stable, exhale. Next, lift your arms to join your chest.

You can keep them at your heart's level if that is what you like, or you could raise them slightly above your heads to spread them out like a tree branch.

Breathe easily. Imagine yourself as a tree. Be firmly rooted and stand tall.

g. Take a deep breath and then return to Tadasana

h. Perform the same circuit, placing the left right on your right thigh.

Benefits: -

This pose will give you a sense grounding and balance. It strengthens your ankles as well as your legs and back. It is a great way to stretch the entire body from head and toe. It increases balance and concentration and calms the mind.

.

Virbhadrasana - Warrior Pose 1

In Sanskrit, Vir means warrior, courageous; Bhadra - auspicious.

Indian mythology, Virabhadra is the name of this pose. There are 3 possible forms for this pose. This is the first.

These are the steps to practicing asana

a. Stand straight on the floor.

b. Spread your legs to about four feet apart.

c. Without moving your left foot, turn your right foot to the side 90 degrees.

d. Do not move your left foot, but turn your body towards the right.

e. Move your arms towards your face and bring both your arms up in front. Then, slowly lift your right knee so that your thigh is parallel to the floor.

f. Take deep, easy breaths.

g. Breathe deeply and get back to your original standing pose.

h. Next, repeat the circuit on the other leg.

Benefits: -

This pose increases balance, concentration, and strength. This pose also strengthens and tones your arms, legs, and lower back. It also energizes the "manipura", which is the third chakra.

Padahastasana - Standing Forward Fold

In Sanskrit, Pada means foot; hasta means hand. This pose refers to hands next to your foot.

These are the steps to practicing asana

a. Standing on your mat with your feet close together, place your hands on your sides.

b. Relax your body. Take a deep breath and slowly raise your arms.

c. You should stretch your body beyond the waist.

d. Breathe deeply and start from your waist. Then, bend forward until your palm rests on the ground.

e. You don't have to touch the ground with your palm first. Relax until you are comfortable.

f. Now, take a deep breath and hold this pose.

g. Stress relaxation for the back.

h. Slowly bring your body up by inhaling.

i. Start with two rounds of practice, and gradually increase the time you hold the pose.

Benefits: -

This pose helps to nourish the brain cells and calm the mind. It also energizes your whole body. It can also improve digestion and metabolism as well increase flexibility in the spine, hamstrings, and back.

Your Daily Yoga Workout

To create an integrated yoga practice for every day of your week, you can mix and match the pranayamas and asanas. It is possible to start by doing each one separately. You can also do it one at a time.

Start practicing and then keep at it. You will be more flexible and more proficient as you practice.

Allow yourself to include 5-10 asanas (mudras) and pranayamas into your daily life to get you started. If you aren't happy with them, increase them or change them. Even if the meditation is only for a couple of minutes, my personal preference is that I begin and end each day's yoga practice with meditation.

You can use the suggested workout as a guide. You can choose to do different poses each day or to follow a specific sequence for a few weeks before changing to the next.

Monday

Bhramari Prnayama

Tadasana or Mountain Pose

Virbhadrasana - Warrior Pose

Padahastasana (or Standing Forward)

Bhujangasana or Cobra Pose

Setu Bandha Sarvangasana or Bridge Pose

Shishuasana, or Child Pose

Meditation for 5 Minutes

Tuesday

Anulom Vilom

Tadasana or Mountain Pose

Vrikshasana / Tree Pose

Utkatasana / Chair Pose

Sukhasana Prithvi Modra

Setu Bandha Sarvangasana or Bridge Pose

Makarasana / Crocodile Pose

Shavasana, or Corpse Pose with Gyan Mudra

Meditation for 5 Minutes

Wednesday

Deep Breathing with Kapalbhati

Vrikshasana (or Tree Pose)

Tadasana or Mountain Pose

Vajrasana (or Thunderbolt) pose

Ardha Matsyendrasana or Half Spinal Twist

Makrasana - Crocodile Pose

Bhujangasana or Cobra Pose

Shavasana, or Corpse Pose

Meditation for 5 Minutes

Thursday

Anulom Vilom

Tadasana or Mountain Pose

Utkatasana / Chair Pose

Padahastasana (or Standing Forward)

Setu Bandha Sarvangasana or Bridge Pose

Viparita Karani and Legs Up The Wall Pose

Shavasana, or Corpse Pose with Gyan Mudra

5 minute meditation in Sukhasana in Prithvi Modra

Friday

Tadasana or Mountain Pose

Utkatasana / Chair Pose

Shavasana, or Corpse Pose

Setu Bandha Sarvangasana or Bridge Pose

Viparita Karani and Legs Up The Wall Pose

Bhujangasana or Cobra Pose

Paschimottanasana or Forward Bend

Shishuasana/Child Pose in Gyan Mudra

5 minute meditation in Sukhasana in Prithvi Modra

Saturday

Sukhasana in Gyan Mudra

Bhujangasana or Cobra Pose

Setu Bandha Sarvangasana or Bridge Pose

Ardha Matsyendrasana or Half Spinal Twist

Vrikshasana or Tree Pose

Virbhadrasana - Warrior Pose

Padahastasana (or Standing Forward)

Tadasana or Mountain Pose

Vajrasana and Thunderbolt poses

Bhramari Prnayama

Meditation for 5 Minutes

Sunday

It could very well be a Meditation Day. Start with deep conscious breathing for 1 minute.

Next, you will need to do Kapalbhati and Anulom Vilom for the next 10 minutes. Then, meditate for 10 minutes in Sukhasana using Prithvi Modra.

It is my preference to do my meditation with mantra. It's just my personal preference. It is possible to meditate by taking your breath in and visualization - whatever works for you.

My personal favourite mantras include:

a. Sanskrit Mantra: - AUM/OM

A powerful universal sound that heals, energizes, and energizes our minds and bodies.

b. Sanskrit Mantra: - SO HUM

So hum refers to I am that. "So," on inhalation, and "hum," on exhalation

"I am strong, fearless, healthy, happy, in bliss, peaceful."

PRANAYAM'S HISTORY

Pranayama and yoga have been around for more than 3000 years. All the intricate techniques and ways pranayama today are a result of simple observation by yogis, rishis, and others who began to observe nature and animals.

They noticed that animals can have different lives depending on how they breath. Based on their observations, they discovered that breathing in a certain manner can have an impact on the health of a particular area of the body. In addition to this, the way that we breathe influences how we feel. And the way that we feel impacts the way our breath. The above statement can be observed by anyone, even yogis. You can see that when you are stressed, your breathing is shallow and fast. If you are calm, your breathing tends to be deep and long.

Simple observations like these, when multiplied over thousands of generations, can be a very powerful tool to help us become physically, mentally, and emotionally healthier.

EVOLUTION and THE TIME LINE OF PRANAYAM

Let's now have a close-up look at which time period pranayama or yoga was documented. The above-mentioned time line can help you see how pranayama has changed over time from simple breathing to advanced breathing exercises. It will also assist those who want to dig deeper into the subject matter, since we will be referring to books in each period.

CIRCA 3000 CE

As early as 3000 BCE, prana was mentioned as a concept in the book names ChandoguyaUpanishad. It talks about the benefits and significance of pran but not pranayama. This could be due to pranayama being a new concept or still in development. Pranayama, which was based on the idea of prana as a vital component of the human body, was established.

CIRCA 1000 BCE

BrihadaranyakaUpanishad is the first text to mention pranayama. This book explains how different breathing techniques can have different effects. Although details regarding the benefits and how to practice pranayama weren't given, they highlight the fact that the practice of pranayama is not new.

CIRCA 10 BCE

We can also find references to pranayama in this period of time, which is a practice for improving physical and psychological health. It emphasizes the fact that we can gain control of our senses by using conscious inhaling, retention of breath, and exhaling. This will eventually lead us to spirituality.

CIRCA 4 BCE

We're introduced to pranayama, yoga and the whole of Maitrayaniya in this time. Yoga was presented in this book as a 6-limb system where pranayama was the greater component. According to this book, 6 limbs make up yoga.

1 Pranayama / Breathing Exercise

2 Pratyahara/ Sensitivity withdrawal

3 Dharana/Concentration

4 Dhyana/ Meditation

5 Tark/Reasoning

6 Samadhi/Union

CIRCA 400CE

Pranayama (or Yoga) was created and documented during this time period by Maharishi Patanjali. He is also the one who expanded yoga from a 6-limb concept to Maitrayaniya and made it a 8-limb concept.

The 8 limbs are

1 Asana/Physical position and exercise

2 Yama / Social precept

3 Niyama/ Ethical precept

4 Pranayama/Breathing Exercise

5 Pratyahara/Sensory withdrawal

6 Dharana/Concentration

7 Dhyana/ Meditation

8 Samadhi/Union

PRANAYAM HAS OVERALL PERSONAL BENEFITS

Regular practice of pranayama can have many health benefits both mentally and physically.

Below is a list od the most common mental benefits of pranayama

It is a great way to reduce stress

- It increases oxygen supply to the brain, which results in improved cognitive performance.

Pranayama, which we do regularly, eventually leads us to meditate quite easily.

Pranayama helps to curb cravings for alcohol, smoking, and other substances.

- It increases emotional well-being by releasing dopamine, oxytocin and dopamine.

- Some cases show that it can help with trauma and PTSD.

Here are some of the most well-known physical benefits.

It can improve the quality of our sleep, and it is extremely effective in tackling insomnia.

It helps us to balance our blood pressure.

- It improves overall digestion by improving the functioning and function of entire organs that are related to digestion like the liver, lungs or kidney.

It boosts immunity by increasing blood RBC, WBC and platelets.

It improves the strength of our respiratory system. This helps to prevent common diseases such as cold and flu, as well as other minor conditions like allergies.

- Because it improves the function of our liver, it aids our body with natural detoxification. This can help reduce skin problems and increase our skin health.

PRANAYAMA HAS MANY TYPES

SURYA BHEDANA

Surya Bhedana pranayama refers to a pranayama that increases heat and energy. Surya, or the right nostril of our body, is known as surya-nadi. This is a symbol representing heat and energy. Chandra nadi (left nostril) is a symbol representing the moon. It represents coolness, calm, and heat. In Sanskrit surya can be translated as sun. Bhedana also means to pass through. Surya Bhhedana, in literal terms, means that the sun passes through (the body), and heat is represented in the body.

BENEFITS

* Increase oxygen level

* It kills intestinal worms

* Cools the body less; useful for cool temperatures

* Increase energy level in the body

* Supportive in cough and cold-related issues

* Very helpful for low blood pressure

* Cures gas-related issues

* Improves the efficiency and effectiveness of entire digestive system

* It reduces anxiety, stress and depression.

STEPS

1. Sit in a comfortable position

2. Now, we need to close our left nostril

3. Now inhale from the right nostril

4. Now close your right nostril, and open your left.

5. Now exhale out of the left nostril

6. You can repeat step 2 to 6 for at most 5 minutes

MOORCHA PRANAYAMA

Moorcha pranayama - This is an advanced pranayama and is not suitable for beginners. Moorcha is Sanskrit means to faint. As you can see, this pranayama causes lightheadedness. If you feel fainting or dizziness, stop pranayama immediately. Although this sounds scary, it can actually improve mental abilities.

BENEFITS

It produces a feeling of euphoria

It enhances mental efficiency

* It boosts positive emotions like joy and cheerfulness.

* It decreases negative emotion like fear, anxiety or frustration

* It prepares for meditation sessions that are effective

STEPS

1. Sit in a comfortable position

2. Relax all parts of your body and spine.

3. Breathe for 5 sec

4. Turn the head slightly to the back.

5. This position should be held for around 5 seconds

6. Take a deep inhale, and hold for 5 seconds.

7. Now move the head into a normal position

8. Repeat steps 3 to 7, approximately 5 times

KAPALBHATI

Kapalbhati is two of the most important pranayama, apart from anulom Villom. If we look at the 80-20 principle, these two pranayamas make up more than half of all pranayama. This is because anulom Vilom has significant effects on brain and nervous systems, and kapalbhati a great impact on digestion and reproduction system. It is recommended that pranayama be performed for 5 minutes each if someone is too busy to do any kind of pranayama.

Kapalbhati is a combination kapal, which refers to the forehead, and bhati that means shining. In other words, kapalbhati literally means shining forehead. This name is apt because kapalbhati can have a significant impact on the digestive system in particular liver and intestine. This allows for the removal of accumulated toxins, which results in better skin health, especially facial skin.

For beginners, it may be difficult to practice kapalbhati over a period of more than one minute. This is because of pain in the abdominal area. These symptoms will disappear over time with regular practice. The initial pain is normal and is part of the healing process. We shouldn't worry too much about it.

BENEFITS

It slows down the aging process

* This helps to reduce acne when used for a long time

* It prevents hair falls

* It helps prevent premature hair greying

It helps to reduce acidity or gas

* It is useful in asthma

* It can help reduce your sinus problem

It can improve skin glow and skin health.

* It improves digestion, absorption and metabolism of food

It improves the functioning of liver & kidneys.

* Helps to balance blood sugar with the aid of pancreas

* It improves energy levels.

STEPS

1. Sit in a comfortable position

2. Inhale deeply

3. Now exhale forcefully and with a stroke

Inhale and push your belly inwards. It should take less then a sec. Because inhalation is automatic, it's important to focus only on exhaling.

4. Step 3

This pranayama should only be done by beginners. It is best to keep it at 1 min for intermediate practitioners. 5 minutes for intermediate practitioners. 15 minutes for advanced practitioners.

DIRGA PRANAYAM

Dirge pranayama has the highest power for the body. Contrary to other pranayamas that involve one part or more of the body in the breathing process this pranayama uses three. These three parts are: 1) Lower belly region (i.e. From the navel downwards, you will find 2 lower chest areas and 3 lower throats. The pranayama involves breathing in and out through various parts of the body. It is a wonderful exercise for all the internal organs.

The pranayama can be practiced by anyone who feels very energized, as it is believed to originate all of the body's internal organs.

BENEFITS

* It makes us very active

* It increases awareness and concentration

* It helps us be at peace and calm.

* It helps reduce stress and anxiety

* It improves the overall functioning and ability of the lungs

PROCESS

There are three parts to the dirga pranayama process

PART1

1. Breathe while expanding your belly.

2. Now exhale and contract the stomach region.

PART2

1. Breathe while expanding your belly.

2. After filling your belly area,

3. Take a few more deep breaths while expanding the lower chest.

4. Now exhale and contract your lower chest.

5. Now exhale and contract the belly region.

PART3

1. Breathe while expanding your belly.

2. You can inhale slightly more to expand the lower chest region.

3. Take a deep breath to expand your upper chest or lower throat.

4. Now inhale as you contract your upper chest.

5. Now exhale while contracting your lower chest.

6. Now contract your belly area so you can exhale all the air out of your body.

This completes all of the dirge pranayama.

Praying this pranayama for a maximum of 1-10 cycles is the preferred number

CHANDRA BHEDANA

Chandra Bhedana pranayama or Chandra Chandra is a very pranayama. It is similar to anulom Vilom pranayama. Chandra is Sanskrit for "moon" and bhedana refers to passing or perceiving through. Our left nostril is known as Chandra nadi and is a symbol of coolness. The right nostril, surya nadi, represents hotness. Chandra Bhadana pranayama means "the moon penetrating within our body". This is the increase in body coolness. This pranayama actually increases the body's cooling. This pranayama would be highly beneficial to anyone living in extremely high temperatures.

BENEFITS

It helps to lower the body's heat

* It can help us lower our temperature during fever

* It reduces negative emotions such as stress, anxiety, anger, etc

* It calms the mind.

STEPS

7. Sit in a comfortable position

8. Now, close the right side of your nose.

9. Now inhale from the left nostril.

10. Now close your left nostril, and open your right.

11. Now exhale out of the right nostril

12. You can repeat step 2 to 6 for at most 5 minutes

BHRAMRI PRANAYAM

Bhramri pranayama has a special quality. Because we need to emit a specific sound when performing this pranayama, the uniqueness of it is due to its nature. This sound is very close to the humming sounds of bees. According to Sanskrit, the sound of bees humming is called "bhramar" in Sanskrit. This pranayama is therefore rightfully called "bhramri", which literally means "like bees humming". This sound can make some people feel nervous, but it is completely worth it.

BENEFITS

* It can increase positive emotions such peace and confidence

* It lowers anxiety, stress, anger, and other negative emotions

* It helps to maintain normal blood pressure

* It's very beneficial for the overall functioning of the heart

* It increases the quality of your sleeping experience

STEPS

1. Sit in a comfortable position

2. Close eyes

3. With the thumb, close both ears

4. We can spread fingers all over the face.

5. Now inhale slowly and deeply through the nose.

6. Now exhale. You should exhale while making a hmmmmmm sound. If it sounds like hummingbees, it is done correctly

You can practice this pranayama anywhere from once to ten times, depending on how comfortable you are.

BHASTRIKA PRIANAYAM

Bhastrika pranayama, also known as Bhastrika pranayama, is best known for creating energy and heat within the body. This is the best pranayama if you are feeling very tired, sick or tired. It generates heat, energy, and helps to overcome fatigue and laziness. If someone feels hot, they should avoid it. This is because it increases pitta doshas. You should try it if you suffer from kaph donsh and vat. It should be completed in no more than 2 minutes.

BENEFITS

* It revitalizes the body, mind, and spirit

* It aids in respiratory problems like the flu and sinuses.

* It increases oxygen in brain

* It increases immunity

It cleanses the liver.

* It can tone the abdominal area

It helps to calm the mind

STEPS

1. Sit in a comfortable position

2. Slowly and deeply inhale through your nose. Next, fill your lungs with air.

3. Now take a deep breath and exhale.

While it is preferable to do this in moderate speed for approximately two minutes, it is better to do it at about 30 secs to one minute for beginners.

BAHYA PRANAYAMA

Bahya pranayama (deep breathing) is a form of pranayama. Baahya (which means outside) is what gave rise to the term bahya. We follow three simple steps in this pranayama: 1 fast exhalation, slow exhalation, and 3 retention. The pranayama bahya was created because we need to keep our breath outside for a longer time. The ratio of inhalation to exhalation should be 2:1. Therefore, if we inhale 3 sec, we should exhale 6 sec, hold our breath for 9 seconds, and then inhale again for 3 sec.

BENEFITS

* Better digestion

* It balances the insulin production and helps to control diabetes

* Increases blood flow to the abdomen.

* Body becomes lighter when unwelcome gas is released

* This pranayama has an external retention section that aids in concentration.

STEPS TO DO

1. Sit in a comfortable position

2. Inhale deeply and fast, preferably 3 seconds

3. Breathe slowly and deeply, at least 6 seconds

4. Now take a deep breath, preferably for 9 seconds. Then pull the area under the navel.

5. Repeat steps 1 to 4, approximately 10 times

Important is to notice that inhalation exhalation should equal retention of breath at 1:2:3.

ANULOMVILOM

Apart from kapalbhati and anulomvilom, pranayama for anulomvilom are the two most important. Pranayama is vital if you want to live healthy lives. The pranayama's main effect is on the 2 hemispheres and the entire nervous network. This is crucial because it involves controlling and regulating pranashiti, the vital energy flowing through nadis, especially ida nadi pingla nadi. Sushumna nadi (controlling prana shakti) is a way to stimulate central nadi. This is a way to detoxify free radicals, toxins, and ida from pingla-nadis. It ultimately results in optimal functioning of both the brain's 2 hemispheres and the nervous system that spreads throughout the body.

BENEFITS

It detoxifies entire nadis

The body is able to remove toxins

It is a great way to fight negative emotions, such as depression and stress anxiety.

It improves lung function.

It aids in Asthma symptoms

This helps maintain normal blood pressure

This is an effective remedy for migraine pain

Balances 3 doshas (i.e. Vat Pitta and Ka

STEPS

1. Sit in a comfortable position

2. Close your right nostril and thumb with right hand

3. Inhale slowly, deeply, from the left nostril. Close the right nostril.

4. Now remove the thumb (right nostril) and close the left nostril.

5. Now exhale out of the right nostril

6. Now, exhale from the right nostril. The left nostril is closed.

7. Now, remove your ring finger from your left nostril.

8. Now exhale from your left nostril. This concludes the cycle of anumolom pranayama.

You can repeat the cycle every minute for a total novice.

Aim to complete the exercise in 5-10 minutes for good health.

The advanced level can complete this task in 15 minutes

AGNI SARA

The words ANGI SARA and AGNI are two words that refer to fire and SARA. This is how we can get the essence of fire by combining these two words.

AGNISARA uses heat to detoxify or cleanse the abdomen. It also helps to maximize the digestive power. All organs of the digestive tract start working at their optimal levels as the detoxification begins. Prana flow rises, which not only increases the energy body but also elevates the mental state and emotional state.

BENEFITS

It reduces anxiety

It strengthens core muscles

It is good for the digestive system.

It builds confidence

It makes us energetic and enthusiastic.

It also increases our determination, resolve, and level of determination

STEPS TO PRACTICE AGNISARA

1 We must stand straight first

2 The distance between the feet should not be wider than our shoulders.

3 We should now bend slightly at the knees

4 We need to now bend our shoulders slightly forward

5 Now place your palm on the thighs.

6 Let's take a few deep breaths in.

7 Inhale slowly, and gradually, until the lungs become completely empty. We should now exhale slowly and smoothly, pulling the abdomen muscles until the navel is in line with the spine.

8 Now we need to hold our breath in that situation

9 Now, we should repeat steps 6-8 5 times if someone is new to the process. We should do this about 10 times for someone who has been practicing it for a month. If the person is an experienced user, we should do this 30 times.

Health & Healing

Pranayama

Pranayama Science

Pranayama, which is itself the science and art of breathing, can be described as Pranayama. Pranayama includes many mechanisms, particularly important organs such the heart or brain. The importance of breathing in a regular rhythm is also important. You can do this by focusing your attention on three steps of breathing: exhaling/inhaling and retaining. Controlling these three aspects of breathing is key to breath control.

Pranayama is technically based in its practice. Pranayama requires one to be able to hold certain positions and also use different breathing techniques. The book will cover many of these practices. However, we will be focusing first on Pranayama's effect on the human internal system (Figure 5) along with the improvement of overall health.

Figure 5.

Human Internal Systems

Yoga teachers, doctors, and spiritual leaders all know the benefits of breath control on the inner system. Therefore, some doctors suggest that patients begin Yoga practices as a form for therapy.

Pranayama, the Endocrine System

When the body harnesses its vitality, it can balance out human hormones. Figure 6 shows how the endocrine (or glandular) system is organized. These glands help the body to perform its functions properly.

Pranayama can therefore improve the functioning of these glands. Pranayama is also known to reverse the signs of aging. This is done by naturally replacing and repairing worn-out' hormones.

Figure 6

The hormones produced by glands in your endocrine system control growth, metabolism, and stress response. Pranayama can help you relax by balancing your breathing and the circulation to various glands responsible.

Your body's reaction to stress changes dramatically when you keep your endocrine and hormonal systems in control. Combine Pranayama with other Yoga practice, such as Asana. It's even better!

Pranayama for Cardiovascular System

The cardiovascular system (see Figure 7) is responsible for transporting oxygen, as well as a host other nutrients, throughout the body.

Pranayama provides more oxygen and reduces cellular wastes. Numerous deaths have resulted from failures of the circulatory systems and the heart.

Yoga and Pranayama are meant to decrease blood pressure, the heart rate, as well as the frequency of the band. Each cell within the body needs specific amounts of oxygen. Proper breathing techniques allow for the regulation and transport of oxygen to all cells.

Figure 7

Yoga allows the body to relax and eliminate stress.

Pranayama for the Respiratory System

Figure 8 shows how the lungs of the respiratory tract are responsible for taking in oxygen and returning carbon dioxide from the outside environment. They form part of the core of human existence along with other respiratory organs. When the lungs cease working, life ceases.

Figure 8

Breathing exercises can therefore be beneficial for the operation of the respiratory tract. The alveoli open, which allows oxygen in greater amounts. Through proper breathing exercises, the diaphragm also becomes stronger. Pranayama helps to eliminate all pollutants around the lungs, and it also releases them from any blockages.

Pranayama to the Digestive System

Figure 9. Indigestion, one of many problems the digestive system is faced with, is one example. Sometimes the faults of our digestive system are what cause many of the health issues that we experience. The digestive system works like an engine and Yoga is a great way to provide all the nourishment that you need.

Figure 9

Pranayama for Musculoskeletal Disorder

Although efficiency of the muscular system during Yoga practices is more closely related to Asana and Pranayama than it is with Yoga, breathing techniques that can be used in any position are important for achieving the desired result. You can lower blood lactate levels by practicing breathing exercises.

Figure 10

Pranayama on Nervous Systems

The nervous system consists of the brain and the spinal cord. We also have the cranial and spinal neural nerves. Figure 11 shows the hierarchy of this system. Figure 12- shows the nervous network in the body. By controlling your breathing, you can control the nervous system. The benefits of breathing exercises are a source of joy and freedom.

Figure 11

Because there aren't equal amounts of air in each nostril, the brain remains disorientated. Pranayama is able to free the brain of any form of obstruction by creating balance in breathing in both nostrils. When this balance is achieved the mind can relax.

Figure 12

Pranayama for Self-healing

Pranayama can help you on your journey to self-healing. Breath acts as a remedy for the body and the mind. It is "life before life". Yoga itself is another type of healing. Pranayama makes it easy to be your own physician with only one pill.

Did you know that the emotions you feel at any given moment can influence your breath? Your emotions can affect your breathing. Being able to control your breath is key to controlling your emotions. To achieve this, you must practice deep, full breathing. Visualize yourself as the bright woman in Figure 13.

Figure 13

Here's a simple guide that will show you how to self heal with Pranayama.

Anuloma Viloma Pranayama Technique for Self-Healing

Yuval Samburski describes Pranayama, a method for self healing, as follows:

With your head up, sit in a comfortable chair that allows you to erect your spine. Dhyana mudra (the mudra of wisdom) is where you place your index finger and thumb on your left thigh. Dhyana mudra dilates bronchi and increases oxygen carrying capability of red blood cell. It also improves concentration.

Figure 14

Right arm lifted, right elbow bent, elbow in air. Your thumb should be folded in half. If folding the index fingers and middle fingers is not easy, hold them straight. Place their tips in the middle of your forehead just above the eyebrows. Close your eyes.

Close your right nostril. Now inhale strongly through the left nostril. Now, inhale from the right nostril. Next, close the left and inhale hard through the right. Finally, close the right nostril to close the right. Exhale out through the left. This was the final round. You can go faster, slower or both. As long as your inhale is full and vigorous, it's okay.

Begin by doing two sets of twenty rounds. In between, you can take a moment to rest or observe. You might find sitting and observing the exercises the most important part. Don't rush. You can do another ten rounds every week. Each set should not exceed two sets total. Do less than you think, but do not do more.

This exercise is intense. If you feel dizzy and/or if something doesn't feel right, take a rest. Then, go back to the beginning.

Anuloma Viloma is a powerful oxygenator that delivers large amounts to the heart and brain. It clears the sinuses, improves the immune system, lowers cholesterol levels, and eliminates headaches (as prevention, don't do it while suffering from migraines!). It vibrates the brain and hearts, providing clarity and fighting depression. It promotes inner peace and bliss. This makes you feel happy inside.

Mind-Body healing

Pranayama's many benefits are innumerable. You may be astonished at how Pranayama is able to affect our emotional and physical beings. Pranayama, which is known for bringing peace and calm to the human spirit, can also be used to heal the body.

Foul emotions put your mind in a panic state and cause you to think very badly. It's not unusual to find people who make bad decisions because of this distortion of their mind.

Figure 15.

But, as a practitioner, the control of your breathe helps you to achieve a calm mind and body. Figure 15 illustrates how balance may feel in your body. The Chakras regulate thought and emotions.

Proper breathing allows for us to communicate more with the muscles, tissues, and organs in our diaphragm than the ones in our chest. This calm state allows for a feeling of security, which in turn makes it easy to engage in other Yoga practices like meditation. Meditation can't be successful if it isn't in a calm state.

Pranayama is a stress- and anxiety-reducing practice.

Pranayama helps you to manage stress and anxiety. This should not happen in a rush, it should be something that lasts for several days.

Here are some basics to help you manage stress and anxiety.

The Balanced Breathing technique:

This is also known to be Sama Vritti. You need to lay down on your stomach.

Now close your eyes and concentrate on your breathing. You can stay in this position for a long time.

You can then inhale by counting up to 4 and exhale, using the exact same count. Be sure to keep your exhalations in the same length.

Once you have been practicing this technique for some time, you will need to achieve higher numbers until you begin to experience an unmistakable sense of relaxation in your body.

Abdominal Breathing

Stress makes it difficult to breathe properly, just like I said about breathing. Adham Pranayama (abdominal breathing) puts you in a better mental state.

Place your face forward and lie down. Place your hands on each side of your stomach. You can also do the same thing as before, but close your eyes. Focus on your breath until your awareness is complete.

This is the idea behind pushing a large amount of your air into your stomach. It will cause your stomach to rise.

Your stomach will rise under your palms when you inhale. Inhaling will cause your stomach to rise under your palms. Exhale and it will return to its previous state. You can repeat this for about ten seconds.

Pranayama is a technique that can be used to treat sleep disorders and insomnia

Sometimes it is difficult to go to bed at night or even at all. Insomnia can result from stress, or other issues in one's private life. It's often something we find difficult to handle. These things result in many sleepless nights and/or waking up earlier than normal when we try to fall asleep. See Figure 16.

Figure 16

The Left Nostril Breathing Technique

This is a breathing technique where the practitioner needs to exhale from his left nostril. The right thumb will block the right nostril.

After that, you will breathe through the left nostril. Keep your eyes shut.

Keep at it for as long you can until your mind and body feel calm.

Relaxing Breathing Technique 7-2-11

In fact, the numbers 7, 2, 11 and 11 are different counts for breathing.

Inhalation consists of seven counts. After holding the breath, you inhale for two counts. Next, exhale for eleven counts.

Continue to do so until your nervous system is calmed down and you feel comfortable going to bed.

Breathing properly and controlling your breath will help you release stress and other negative emotions from your body. It allows you to put aside all your worries and focus on your breath.

"Breathing has the dual nature that it is both voluntary (and also compulsory).

autonomic. That is why the breathing illuminates the eternal query about what we can control, change or not.

~ Leslie Kaminoff

Anatomy Of The Breath

Understanding Our Breath

We all know that breathing is important for our survival, but we don't always realize that breathing is an interesting activity and can have a conscious connection to it.

Many people don't realise that air is passing from their nostrils down into their lungs. When you pay attention to the details of breathing, you can actually feel them all. Pranayama is more effective when you know how to do this as an Yoga practitioner.

Although the art of breath control may appear unconscious on the surface, it is possible to exert complete control over the process. Breath control and awareness are only two steps away from understanding the mechanics of breathing.

Gross Anatomy

To begin our gross anatomy of breathing, we will examine the organs responsible to aid the process. This is in an effort to give you an understanding and recognition of the organs.

Breathing organs

The Nose

It is often the nose that is first mentioned when talking about breathing. Maybe you've ever tried to cover both nostrils but suddenly realized that it was impossible to breathe. You might have just learned it through your school years. But the nose is an integral part of the breathing system. It is also more prominent because it's located externally.

We inhale through our noses. It can be found in different sizes and shapes depending on the person. It is also more comfortable for some people to breathe from one nostril rather than the other. You may have also seen the bony structure that separates each nostril.

The sinuses are another important part of the nose and play an essential role in Yoga's breathing process. They are found on both sides and provide air conditioning to the brain. The sinuses help us think clearly and make our heads clearer. Proper breathing can expand the sinuses. This allows enough air to cleanse them and allow them to function normally.

The Pharynx

The pharynx allows air and food to travel from the mouth, nose, and lungs. There are two tubes that connect the ears to nasopharynx. They are called the Eustachian, or auditory tubes. It also includes tonsils, or lumps of lymphatic tissues. When breathing, the tonsils, particularly the adenoids, are crucial. This is because if they become swollen, breath cannot pass through the nasal cavities. Swollen tonsils can lead to crash breathing, where people breathe through their mouth.

Larynx

The larynx (also known as the voicebox) is directly connected to the Pharynx. It's located just below it. It contains the glottis, vocal cords and other components that make sound. The epiglottis allows exhalations to pass through it, which causes the vocal cords and vocal chords to tremble.

Lungs

The lungs are located in the chest. One is on the left, and one on the right. The lobes refer to the different parts of the lung. The lungs transport the air we inhale to the red cells. The lungs regulate the blood's pH. It regulates the amount carbon dioxide present in the body at any time.

Trachea

This organ is also known as the windpipe. This nickname may be a good way to explain the importance of this organ. The trachea is a wide, hollow-like tube measuring approximately 4 inches in length that connects to the lungs. It is responsible in bringing air into and out the body through breathing.

It is made up several rings of cartilage containing moist tissue, called mucosa. The trachea is flexible membrane that contracts and expands during inhalation.

The Mouth

During breathing the mouth serves as an additional airway. This is especially true if we require more air that can pass through our nostrils. This is obvious when you experience panting or gasping for air. Also, when we are experiencing nasal problems or other issues like a common cold, the mouth is required to help us breathe. The practice of mouth breathing is part of certain yogic breathing methods.

How It All Works

All these organs work together in the system. They are interdependent. The importance of each organ must be understood.

Pranayama practice should not include such ideas. You should instead try to bring them together for the best experience in your breath control.

Here's how breathing works inside our bodies.

Inhalation

Inhalation means that you inhale air. The diaphragm contracts during inhalation, causing it downward. Inhalation also opens up the lungs to allow for more airflow, which in turn allows it expand. The air drawn from the mouth or nose travels through your trachea and stops at your lungs. From there it branches into your bronchial tubes and finally into your lungs.

As I stated earlier, the lungs aid in the transfer of oxygen into the red cells. The next step is to carry the oxygen from the air cells into the blood.

Exhalation

This is the act or process of breathing in. This occurs when the diaphragm relaxes and the chest expands. Once the chest starts to contract, which causes less space around this area to contract, carbon dioxide will be pushed from your system through your nose or mouth.

This is a quick way to try the two described processes.

Place your right hand below the sternum. Inhale deeply. Do this for a few times. Then, you inhale. Things begin to fall back the way they were. Your stomach returns to its normal position and your diaphragm moves back up.

The Concept Of Residual Air during Breathing

Adults will likely breathe in and exhale sixteen to seventeen times a minute. Researchers believe that the nose takes in about half a liter of air each minute.

But, not all of the oxygen drawn during breathing leaves your nose. It travels to your lung. There is residual oxygen that remains in each organ (including the nose or mouth, larynx, trachea, and so forth). This residual gas does not participate in exchange of gases.

Researchers also discovered that the deeper the breath is, the greater the residual air. Yogi practitioners often recommend deep breathing for yogic exercises.

Volume and Rates

Respiratory minute volume

Also known as minute ventilation or respiratory minute volume, it is the volume in which air is exhaled and inhaled from an individual's lungs each minute. Volumes of breath often correlate with the amount of carbon dioxide present in the body.

According to scientists, the human body is able to hold approximately five to eight liters (or more) of air every minute. Accordingly, the body is able to regulate the system's homeostasis with respect to these volumes.

Respiratory Rate

Respiratory rate measures how many breaths an individual takes every minute. It is often measured manually by counting the number times that the chest rises in a time period of rest. Adults can take approximately twelve to eighteen minutes to breathe, while those under eleven years of age tend to take more in a single minute.

The quality of a person's emotions and their ability to control the volume and rate of breathing can impact the health. An abnormal rate in respiration can lead to heart and lung disease, anxiety, stress, depression, and even heart attacks. Normal respiration for an individual should range between 12-25. Normal respiration rate is between 12 and 25.

Anything lower or higher than this limit is considered abnormal.

Pranayama yoga breathing exercises are a good way to regulate both your respiratory minute volume as well as your rate of respiration.

The Thoracic Cage

The thoracic cavity, also known by the rib area, covers a portion of the chest. The thoracic area protects vital internal parts located in the abdomen and thoracic regions against outside elements.

It protects the heart and lungs by acting as a bony protector. It contains twelve pairs, twelve pairs, of the sternum, thoracic vertebrae, and coastal cartilages. It is essential for breathing.

Thoracic Cage in Breathing

The thoracic crate aids breathing by using muscles between the inner and outer intercostal cartilages. Inhaling air causes the thorax cavity to expand and the ribs to shoot upward.

Some experts refer to this as the diaphragmatic-rib cage breathing. Because the diaphragm lies in the lower half of the ribs cage. Inhalation stops the stomach from rising by contracting the muscles at the front of your abdomen.

The stomach then presses against the bottom of diaphragm. This causes the bottom to lift and the rib cage also to lift. During this time, the ribs are displaced from the body, which broadens the lungs, and expands the thoracic cavity.

Muscles to Breathe

The muscles responsible to breathing are just as important than the organs. These muscles are also known to be the breathing pump muscles. These muscles form the semi-rigid bellows which surround the lungs.

The expansion or compression of the thoracic cavity is also a responsibility for the respiratory muscles. The inspiratory and expiratory muscles are the muscles that control the expansion and then inhalation. The respiratory muscles are listed below.

The Diaphragm

The major muscle for inhalation, the diaphragm, is located at the diaphragm. It connects to the lower and lumber vertebrae in your spinal cord. During contraction, diaphragm expands and descends into the abdomen.

It uses its dome-like structure to finally separate the thoracic from the abdominal cavities. The diaphragm is able to aid in vomiting and defecation. It does this by pressing on the abdominal cavity.

Intercostal Muscles

The area between the 12 pairs of ribs is where the intercostal muscle are found. The intercostal muscle can be located either inside the ribs' inner surfaces or outside the ribs' surface. These muscles allow for certain movements, such as pulling, pushing, lifting or lifting.

Expiration (Exhalation). Muscles

Exhaling requires less energy to perform than inhalation. This means that the muscles can function with less effort. They are most commonly found near the abdominal wall.

Pranayama is an example of deliberate breathing. This means that the muscles are more functional, and they tend to push the diaphragm into thoracic space. The exhalation becomes voluntary when the lung or rib cage is tired.

Breathing Mechanisms & Pulmonary Function

Pulmonary respiration is comprised of mechanical actions that create an interplay between the lungs, the external environment, and the lungs. Inhalation is when oxygen is drawn into your body. Exhalation is when carbon dioxide is exhaled out. The difference in pressure between the atmosphere (lung) and the airway is responsible for the way that breathing works.

To be able to breathe in pulmonary mode, your chest must be able expand and contract during the process. Because the lungs are not equipped with muscles, it is unable to start any volume changes. The lungs take cues from the chest's movement and follow it.

Because the pressure in the air outside is much higher that the intrapulmonary pressure, it travels through your lungs to take in oxygen. To allow gases to exchange within the system, it is necessary to change the intrapulmonary tension.

Subtle Anatomy: The Five Pranas

Although we've briefly covered the five major Pranas here in the first Chapter, we'll be going into greater detail in this Chapter. Prana, like we mentioned earlier, can be described as the life force. Prana, however, is often overlooked.

Breathing, both exhaling and inhaling, gives us the ability to control and be aware of the Prana through Yoga. Pranayama allows the individual to release the power, vitality and power of Prana.

Each Prana is a path to light. Vayus is also known for being the "powerful of air". Pranas are said to be in control of every aspect of our bodies as well as our presence.

Apana Vayu

The Apana Vayu can be found in the lower abdomen. This is where all of our fluids and thoughts flow. It ensures that we have a proper elimination of any waste products.

People who experience constipation problems are experiencing difficulties with the Apana vayu's downward movement. As well, there are women who have irregular periods. Apana must be reconciled so these areas can fulfill their duties in the system.

This can be done by breathing down the spine and through the Root Chakra. Then exhale through the bottom part of your body, the legs or the feet. In this way, the individual has an immediate attachment to Earth and a sense of security. People who have been confronted by negative emotions like anxiety, fear, and stress often find relief.

Samana Vayu

This Prana addresses digestion. This is not just about the food or drinks we consume. It also includes abstract things like information we receive from reading news and society or listening to people. Samana vayu issues can lead to indigestion of abstract or emotional foods.

Food can be difficult to digest. When it comes to emotions, many people find themselves unable to forget or reconcile the painful experiences they have had, or even deal with the new bad news.

Samana, when harnessed can help us eat or assimilate what we need. It is also beneficial to our overall well-being and existence.

Prana Vayu

This meaning is distinct from Prana which we commonly refer as "life force" This is concerned with the quality and quantity of food that we consume. It also discusses the mental state we are in at any given time. Do we have the ability to disconnect from our senses, like Pratyahara

The individual may have difficulty focusing on meditation when there are problems with Prana Vayu. This is evident in those who seek out vain things or thoughts that are not necessary for their bodies and minds. Inhaling into "Third Eye" allows the practitioner to achieve this Prana, which is a way to relax the mind and relieve stress. The practitioner could not embark on his internal journey towards freedom until that point.

Udana Vayu

Udana concerns the upper half of the body, and its upward movement. It refers to the physical growth and shrinkage of older people, as well as their physical maturation after leaving childhood. There is a certain amount of mental development when the Udana Vayu is present and stagnancy if it isn't.

People who lack Udana tend not to want to leave a place they've been living for so long, whether it's a job with no prospects of advancement or stability in a few places.

Yoga practitioners with difficulty lifting their heads up or maintaining a straight posture when practicing Yoga will show their deficiency. To bring the Udana to life, you must inhale from the base on the spine all the way up to your throat.

Vyana Vayu

This is Prana of circulation. It allows food to reach all areas where it is needed. People who have a stable Vyana are often able to think clearly and express their thoughts. Vyana Vayu assists the Pranas to function properly because it can reach all areas of the body.

Vyana requires that practitioners inhale into the heart and exhale from their hands.

Pranayama, Yoga, and Pranayama are all about connecting the mind and body to one another.

The Five Sheaths

According to Yoga terminology, the five sheaths represent the five Koshas. Yoga can help us reach a deeper connection with our body, and our minds. For a holistic healing process to occur, it is necessary that the practitioner realizes the five sheaths.

According to the Taittiriya Upanishad yogic literature and yogic writings, each individual is thought to have five sheaths. These sheaths are placed under each other and serve as a shield for the soul. The soul is similar to a gift that has five wrappings. They must all be open before it reaches its destination.

It is important, however, to recognize that even though these layers are deeply embedded in each other they cannot be separated. Events that take place within one sheath will have an immediate effect on other sheaths.

1. The Annamaya Kosha -- The Physical Sheath

This is called the Annamaya Kosha. It is the most perceptible layer of all and, therefore, the one we are the most aware of. If the individual is not a Yoga practitioner, however, she will still be unaware of what is going on in the body.

The physical sheath refers specifically to our bones, muscles, and skin. It's the layer that Yoga practitioners tend to be most focused on. This Kosha can help the individual achieve balance in her body and strength. She begins to notice the importance of what food she eats, and which foods are best for certain areas of her body.

2. Pranayama Kosha is the Energy Sheath

This is Pranayama Kosha. It is only felt unlike Annamaya. Some practitioners may abandon it during Yogic practices. Each sheath is essential if you desire to Yoganasya, or union of mind and body.

Pranayama Kosha is achieved when Asana and Pranayama are combined. It brings the Prana or life-force into the body. Meditation becomes much easier once you become more aware of the breath. The Prana is a way to make an individual feel more energy-efficient through their breathing.

This energy is focused upon controlling the breath. Unstable Prana also means an unstable breath. It is possible to harness the breath and channel it in all the right places, which will bring peace to your mind and help you with the Yoga practices of your eight limbs.

3. The Manomaya Kosha -- The Mental Sheath

The Manomaya Kosha (mental layer) is also known. It allows the individual to reason, think, and imagine many things. It affects the mind as well as the individual's thoughts. This sheath assists the individual in making sense of everything that is happening around him.

But, because we have a difficult time managing certain emotions, some people might find their way into this sheath. Yoga is a way to improve our mental health. Yoga is often a way for people to overcome fear and anxiety that has impacted their decisions in life.

4. The Vijnanamayakosha -- Wisdom Sheath

The Vijnanamaya kosha, or wisdom, stimulates awareness that comes from within. It includes intuition and conscience. This layer has a deeper inner knowing, separate from feelings and thoughts. Yoga has many practices that help to lower the Manomaya Kosha's (mental sheath), so we can listen to our intuition, and then let it guide us to the truth.

5. The Anandamaya Kosha -- The Bliss Sheath

This is Anandamaya Kosha. It is the highest layer among all layers, and it is therefore more easily overlooked by the practitioner than the other. A thorough Yoga practice is required to reach the bliss sheath. It is well worth it. This is because "bliss" can be found in the form of freedom, fulfillment, and a greater understanding of yourself.

A person becomes more aware of her own body and takes pleasure in it. These examples can be found in the joy you feel when you do things such as acting, writing, speaking publically, acting, or painting. What gives you joy? But, until you start a Yoga practice, you might not know about this bliss sheath.

Yoga helps to bring awareness to all the sheaths of your life. It makes your life more meaningful, purposeful and fulfilling. It does not matter how difficult or simple they may seem, it is always a great thing to be aware of all the Koshas.

Chakra Essentials

Chakras, or energetic centers, are where the individual's energy flows through. Chakra is actually Sanskrit for "wheel". It is often called the "wheels for energy throughout your body" in Yoga practice.

The 7 Chakras

Chakra 1

This is the Muladhara. Also known as the Root Chakra. It is located at base of spine, and connects to the skull. It is considered to be the foundation for life and the source of stability. These people have stable feelings, fearlessness, security and are at the root of the Root Chakra.

Chakra 2

This is the Svadhisthana. It is the center of creativity and pleasure. It can be found in the navel, just above the genitals. It allows an individual to enjoy pleasure in many ways. It is particularly useful in sexually related activities. A active Svadhisthana can also help us express our creativity.

Chakra 3

People with active Manipura have a tendency to feel confident and high self-esteem. It is located above your navel and connects directly to your breastbone. The chakra can also be associated with self-worth and positive thoughts.

Chakra 4

The Anahata is the connection chakra between the individual's spirit and his mind. It is located at the center of your chest. This chakra is essential for love. It allows us to feel connected with others, be happy, have compassion and be loved.

Chakra 5

This chakra, known as the Vishuddha or the Vishuddha, allows us to express our deepest truths and communicate them clearly to others. It is located in the throat.

Chakra 6

This is the Ajnachakra. It is located between your eyebrows and the forehead. This is the "third" eye, as Yogis call it. It is the energy center which stimulates intuition as well as inner knowledge. It is often called the "third eyes" because it helps to see the larger picture. The chakra also has wisdom and imagination.

Chakra 7

The Sahaswara Chakra lies at the top and is found on the scalp. If this chakra is activated, we can become enlightened and have a connection with our spirit. It's similar to the last shed where one experiences pure bliss as well as a connection with his or her spiritual self.

The Importance and Value of Our Chakras

The chakras are energy centers that have a connection to major nerve centers throughout the body. Every chakra has nerves, organs. They are also closely linked to the mental condition of the individual. You can see that maintaining their function is crucial for an individual. The chakras can be found in the physical world as well as in the spiritual.

One chakra cannot be disabled while others are too busy. They will not do their job as intended. If energy is blocked from any center, the chakras and associated parts of the body will shut down. This can lead to illness.

Pranayama can help you balance and harmonize all seven chakras.

Breath as Subtle Aatomy

Prana travels through the body, reaching all five sheaths using subtle energy channels known as the Nadis. Nadi is a Sanskrit name for motion. While invisible to the naked eyes, the Nadis act as subtle energy channels and carry the vitality or breath to the individual. They are also able to give strength and power to the heart, allowing for movement.

The Nadis and the nervous system are both closely linked to the Nadis. There are approximately 72,000 Nadis in different parts. Figure 17 shows three major Nadis that Yoga texts agree with.

Figure 17.

Ida

Ida, in Sanskrit, means "comfort". It is associated with the right part of the brain and the left half of the body. It is often connected to the moon's feminine energy and thus lunar energy. It is responsible in carrying life energy which purifies the mind and controls all of one's mental endeavors. Ida is located to the left of Susumna. It stops in the right nostril. It is also associated with the left testicles and male individuals.

Pingala

This Nadi begins at the right end of the Sushumna Nadi. Pingala has been associated with heat and sunlight, while Ida stands for cooling. Pingala flows right through the nose.

It can stay in the nose for up to an hour before returning when the individual is engaged in other activities. It activates left side of brain. Bhedana Pranayama practices are most effective to make this Nadi activate.

Sushumna

The Sushumna Nadi, which runs through the spine, is the connection between the root and the crown chakras. When the breath travels through both nostrils, Sushumna Nadi becomes active. Pranayama exercises can make this happen. As the Sushumna moves across the spine, it indicates that Prana can also move through the other Nadis.

Purification Of The Nadis

Pranayama is the ultimate way to purify your Nadis. It involves inhaling the life energy throughout your body. To start purification, an individual must first adopt an Asana position. Once she is in that position, she will be firm in any other.

To flush out the Sushumna dirt, the person should be in Padmasana (or a comparable comfortable seated position, with a long, straight spine) Pranayama refers to retaining breath. The individual should do this by inhaling the left nostril as long as possible before exhaling the right.

You can repeat the process by inhaling through your left nostril. This process will make the Nadis more active and purified if it is repeated over a time period.

Pranayama (breath-centered asana practice) and Pranayama (pranayama) are two of the best gifts from the Yoga tradition.

Maintain our physiological, metabolic and other health.

Health and well-being

Balance our emotions and clarify our thoughts."

~ Gary Kraftsow

The Practice

Pranayama und Asana

Introduction to Breathing

Breathing can be described as the link between the conscious part and the unconscious. Breathing is the act that unites the mind with the body. The act of bringing about a union between the mind and the body at the most basic level for an average person - someone who isn't interested in Yoga - breathing can be considered an involuntary action that the individual doesn't believe she should be aware.

However, she is unaware that breathing is the way to freedom, a clear mind, better mental health, and overall action which can be affected by one's conscious actions.

Costal Breathing

This type of breathing involves movement of the ribs in order to enhance both exhalation (and inhalation) during breathing. The intercostal muscle (both the internal and external intercostals), and the spinal erectors, are both responsible for costal breathing. This breathing process allows one to focus on all the edges of the spine by compressing it during exhalation and expanding it during inhalation.

Costal breathing has another benefit for the person: it gives her consciousness even without her ribcage.

Costal Breathing Exercises

Costal breathing exercises help to develop certain postures such as the neck, chest, and ribs.

Exercise 1: you must be in a slump. Begin by sitting cross-legged across the floor. Allow your head to dangle forward with your ribcage pushing backwards. Or, stand straight.

Standing, you can perform the same actions as sitting. However you will need to arch your knees slightly so you form an S shape.

Let your pelvis move backwards while you slump. Your spine will bend forwards to give it a rounder shape. Your head should be dangled forward towards your stomach.

Your spine may appear stretched as a result. This is because the lumbar spine gets pushed forward. It is possible to feel your neck being pressured. In the end, your ribs should point downwards.

After you have gotten into a comfortable sitting position, lift your head up and stop arching. Your pelvis should move forward to align your lumbar spine. Keep your head facing up. Your chest should be open, and you should feel the straightening in your neck.

The actual sensation of breathing begins once you are standing tall. Inhale. Begin by inhaling. Next, shift your head towards the back and upwards. It is not necessary to pull your neck forwards. After exhaling, relax. Then, relax your shoulders and neck as you move the ribs towards the pelvis. These areas should be felt, including the waist. Your breathing will become easier as you try to get these parts to work together.

While you are doing the exercise, focus on the front area of the ribcage. Inhaling through the nose will raise your ribs, allowing you to focus on the front of your ribcage. As a consequence, the spaces between the pairs ribs become larger. Exhalation causes the ribcage to be reduced as slow as possible.

It is possible to also open the rear end of the ribcage with coastal breathing exercises.

Exercise 2: This is the simpler of the two. As much air as possible. While you are doing this, feel the air rising to the back of your ribs.

If you let go of the breath, the back of your ribs will begin to move downward. As a result, your chest is expanding more than your back. Breathing into your rear ribcage will allow you to draw in more air.

Costal Breathing is all based on using the ribs when breathing. The effects of breathing can change the shape and size of the ribcage. This allows the individual to have control over her ribcage. Also, it provides a basis for diaphragmatic respiration.

Diaphragmatic Breathing

As stated earlier, breathing is primarily performed by the diaphragm. Blood oxygenation requires diaphragmatic breath. Also, diaphragmatic breathing helps the diaphragm muscles gain strength and regulate the rate of respiration.

Being able to breathe from your diaphragm will help you save more energy. Diaphragmatic breathing causes the lungs to expand, allowing them to draw in more oxygen.

As we get older, our ability to correctly breathe is affected. Infants are able to involuntarily use the diaphragm to do this. In this way, an average person might draw in their breath from the chest rather than the diaphragm.

Diaphragmatic Breathing exercises

Exercise 1: Lie flat on a surface with your back facing the ceiling. Your head should be supported by a pillow. Now, bend your knees. As well as supporting your knees with a pillow, you could also use one.

Placing one hand on the top of your chest and the second in the area under the ribs, place the other. This is to help you feel your diaphragm in the air you inhale and exhale.

Once your hands are properly placed and your head and knee support are supported, start to draw in air slowly through the nostrils.

Your stomach pushes your palm forward when you breathe in air. Keep your other hand in your chest.

Relax your stomach muscles and allow them to contract. Now, exhale and press your lips against the air.

Exercise 2: For this exercise, you must sit down in a chair. Place your back on a chair or sofa so that you feel as comfortable as possible. You can also bend your knees as in the first exercise and rest your head and shoulders against a chair.

Place one hand on your chest in the upper area, and the second hand below your rib cage. Once you've placed your hands where they belong, with your head supported and your knees supported by the other hand, start to draw in as much air as you can through the nostrils.

Your stomach pulls your hand forward while you inhale. But, keep your other hand on the chest.

Relax your stomach muscles and allow them to contract. Now, exhale and press your lips against the air.

Exercise 3: To finish this technique, find a leather belt and wrap the belt around your rib cage. This allows for the diaphragm (the major muscle that helps you breathe) to be involved in the process.

Fix the belt around your bottom by wrapping it around your ribs. You can then take deep breaths through your nose as the belt wraps around you.

Diaphragmatic breathing is a way to keep your mind still. You can count backwards or forwards each time you breathe in or out. This allows you focus only on breathing and keeps your mind off of everything else.

The Valsalva Method

The Valsalva Method, also known by Valsalva maneuver, is a way to exhale air forcefully when there is a blockage in the airway. Some people use this technique without realizing it. This is the case when someone sneezes but tries to hold it back. However, this practice can help one gain strength in Yoga and fitness.

It is common to use the Valsalva method for breathing to increase breath holding while weight training. It is crucial because not all weight trainers can hold their breath correctly. This technique helps them learn to breathe correctly even though their nostrils are closed.

It raises the pressure of air in thoracic cavities and in lugs to force out breath. When the abdominal muscles are hardened, the diaphragm and other organs around this area can squeeze upwards against it.

This upward shoot in the diaphragm causes muscles in the chest to harden. At the same moment, the larynx would close, forcing air to the lungs.

If the individual is trying lift a heavy object, however the Valsalva method may prove to be particularly helpful. For weight lifting, it is a popular method.

Pranayama in Asana

Asana means the posture in which someone is sitting during Yoga. Yoga offers many different postures (Asanas), that allow for meditation. Asanas form a key part of Yoga, as I mentioned previously. Asana does NOT refer to any position. Instead, it refers only to the one that is most convenient and appropriate for the individual so that he can have a seamless connection with his spirit and mind.

Being able to successfully practice Asana requires that the individual control her Prana so that she can channel her subtle energy in the right directions. Pranayama can only be performed by an individual whose posture is most comfortable for her. This shows there is a connection between the two limbs and you cannot do either without the other.

Here are some Asana postures that will help you to perform Pranayama or prepare for meditation.

Padmasana

This pose is also called the Lotus Pose. This is because it involves a lotus-shaped pose. It is considered the most powerful pose, as it allows you to meditate more and pay more attention to your mind.

How to perform Padmasana

The individual should place his legs straight in front and sit on the ground. After that, fold the right knee in half and place it on the left side of the body. Then, place the folded left knee on your right side.

While he is doing this, she should ensure the spine stays straight. To do this, she can raise her torso toward the inner right foot. He can be confirmed by her slight swinging of his leg in a to-and-fro motion.

Now, you can place your hands on each of the knee joints. After that, place your hands on each knee joint.

Figure 18

When you are done, raise your spine and keep your head up. Now, take slow deep breathes in and out through your nose.

Svastikasana

It's not always easy to do Padmasana from the Auspicious pose. This could be because of physical limitations, such as tightened or limited hips or restricted muscles in certain parts of the body. Svastikasana may be less difficult than Padmasana.

How to perform Svastikasana

In a sitting position, erect your back. Spread your legs wide in front of you and fold the left foot. The sole of the right leg should be placed inside the right hip. The right leg can be folded in the opposite direction. Bend it slightly and place your foot between the knee and the calf. Place your wrists on each side of the knee. Now you can inhale and exhale normally. Figure 19.

Figure 19

This position allows for stability and helps one to meditate. This is possible because the body becomes more comfortable and straightened.

Siddhasana

This is also known to be the "perfect" and "accomplished pose. It is next to Padmasana and considered the most important asana of meditation. It helps to maintain a comfortable and straight spine for a long period of time.

Prana can flow in an upward direction toward the spinal column. If a person can hold this position for a prolonged time, she is likely to be able manage her sexual urges.

Siddhasana is how to do it

Your legs should be pressed together. Place the left foot on the floor, with your legs pressed together. If the individual is female, the foot should go in the labia majora. Then, elevate the right leg to place the foot on the labia majora.

Figure 20

Toes should be placed on the right foot. Your knees should remain flat on the ground. Keep your spine straight and focused. Now, take deep, natural inhales.

Savasana

This is also known to be the "corpse", or "corpse" pose. It can be difficult for practitioners to achieve because the individual must relax completely in order to perform this pose.

How to perform Savasana

You will need a flat and comfortable surface. Place your back flat on the surface. Spread your feet apart. With your back to the floor, place your arms on your side. When you are done, close your eyes so you can focus on your breathing.

In this situation, you should breathe from the diaphragm. Continue to inhale and exhale until you feel totally comfortable.

Figure 21

Next, take a deep breath through the nose and straighten your body. Keep your legs elevated as slowly and gently as you can, but don't apply too much pressure to your back. Do the lifting from your calves and/or laps.

Then, lift your arms up from your side and close your fists. Keep this position for as long and as possible. After completing the pose, exhale through your nose to return to a relaxed state.

Pranayama is a practice that requires both stability and mindfulness in order to bring together the two elements. To achieve this, Asana must be stable in order to allow for seamless breathing. I will stress again that the limbs of each limb are interrelated.

Vinyasa, Connecting Breath And Movement

Yoga practitioners are well-known for arranging their movements according to their breath so that it flows from one pose into the next. Vinyasa simply means "to arrange in some unique way". Vinyasa Yoga aims to get the body in a better condition and physical state. This is accomplished by synchronizing the individual's physical movements with his breathing. It allows you to move in different asanas by matching your breathing rhythm with your muscles.

Some Yogis believe that movement and breath can be linked, i.e. Asana that focuses on breath is the most important Yoga exercise. It is easy for people to understand why.

Vinyasa can be practiced in a series of steps. This series of poses is necessary for the individual to learn to connect his breathing and his movement. Vinyasa has a series of sequences that allow you to connect your breath.

Surya Namaskara - The Sun Salutation Sequence

Vinyasa Yoga is incomplete without the sun salutation, as shown in Figure 22. The sun salutation sequence increases oxygen circulation. This sequence is dependent on your ability to breathe properly. It is essential that you can breathe properly. This sequence includes a series of postures that can be used for breathing. You can start your yoga practice by lying down on your Yoga Mat.

1. Mountain pose: To begin, you will need to stand in the mountain position. Keep your feet slightly apart and place your hands sideways. You can also join them in a prayer posture. Then inhale deeply.

2. Let's get your hands up. The next time that you inhale, extend your arms straight up and bend your body as far as you can until you feel it is impossible to stretch your legs.

3. Head to knees.

4. Inhale. Now, push your right leg backwards.

5. Plank pose. Continue inhaling, pushing the left leg forward to create a plank-like position. Continue to maintain this position and inhale.

6. Stick pose. Inhale, and then lower your body to the ground. This will allow you to stretch like you're doing push-ups. Try to keep your feet as flat as possible, but don't let your hands touch the floor.

7. This is the Upward Dog posture. Inhale deeply and move your body toward the front.

Your torso should be lifted with your arms. Also, raise your legs so your feet and hands don't touch the floor.

8. This is known as the Downward Dog. Inhale and raise your hips, ensuring your feet and hands are on the floor. Your hips should be pushed back and forth.

Figure 22

The four remaining postures in this sequence, which are in ascending order, consist of the lunge and mountain poses.

Restorative Therapies

Yoga poses can be used for healing and restoration. These postures help ease stress and allow for relaxation. These postures can be used to help you attain restoration in your Yogic practises.

Balasana

This pose is also known as the Supported child's pose, which can be seen in Figure 23. This requires you to rest your buttocks on your buttocks, and instead sit on your shins. Spread your knees in front of a support device, such as a pillow or a blanket.

Figure 23

Keep the support in front and between your shins. They support the rest your body, from your waist up to the support that has been chosen. You can place your arms on one side of the support while you turn your head regularly towards the other.

Baddha Konasana

This pose is called the Bound Angle Pose. It can be done upright, as shown in figure 24, or forward folded in Figure 25, as shown. This requires you to sit on the floor with your knees outward so that your soles touch each other.

To raise your buttocks, you can only sit on one piece of blanket. You can then fold another blanket under your knees from both sides. Place the desired support, perhaps a pillow, on top of your head. With your head facing downwards, place your arms and head on the support. You should stay in this position as long as possible.

Figure 24

Figure 25

Uttana Shishosana

This is the Puppy pose. Place the support on a flat surface and kneel down in front of it. The support should be placed in the middle of your body, between your waistline and your chest. Move your arms forward and place your head on the other lever just before the support or pillow.

Figure 26

Setu Bandha Sarvangasana

This is the Supported Bridge Pose. The Supported Bridge Pose requires you to lie on your side and bend your knees. Look for a block, and place it between your waistband and your buttocks. The waist will now rise and point forward. Place your hands on the sides of your body, and extend your arms to the side.

To keep your legs together, tie a belt or elastic band around your thighs. This allows for the chest to expand. Continue to hold the position until you find it uncomfortable.

Supta Baddha Konasana

This is Reclining Boundangle Pose. This pose requires you to place support behind your back while you sit on the ground. As you will be lying down on the support, rather than resting your stomach against it, the support should be more powerful than in previous poses.

A belt should be tied around the waist. Pull it into the thighs. Now, raise your knees until the knees are straight up.

Figure 27

Now, lie back down on the support. Wrap the belt around your knees. Place some support underneath your knees. Your eyes should be closed. Turn your head towards the ceiling. You can then keep this position for as long and as you like.

These restorative positions give the mind and body a peace that is unmatched. The organs that are stressed relax and you can focus your attention on the other activities the person would be engaging in.

Yin Yoga Postures

Yin Yoga refers to a special form of Yoga that focuses more on the fascia, joints, tendons, and ligaments than the muscles. It offers poses that are quite distinct from those used in restorative positions, even though both Yogic practices demand that you maintain a pose for long periods of time.

Chinese medical philosophy holds that the elements Yin should be considered calm and static. Yin Yoga emphasizes the connection of the tissues, in contrast to other Yogic practices which focus on movement. Yin Yoga also offers a sense of satisfaction. This is because you are required not to enjoy a pose but you must maintain it.

Here are some Yin Yoga poses you might like to try.

The Snail Pose

Spread your body flat on a surface. You should raise your legs until they are about 90 degrees. Now, stretch your leg until it touches your back. The result is that your lower spine will tilt slightly and only your upper spine will be on the ground.

In certain cases, however the upper spine might tilt toward the side. It all depends on your body's flexibility. For practitioners with flexible bodies, it is easy to raise their foot towards the back of the head. You will want to keep that position for approximately three minutes when you achieve it. See Figure 28.

Figure 28

The Dragon Pose

With your hands and feet, start by crouching on your stomach. Now, place your left foot in the gap between the two fingers and pull the right knee backwards. Place your hands on the forefoot of your knees as support.

Figure 29

Once you are balanced on your left leg, gently lower your right thigh towards the ground. This will stimulate your stomach and spleen. Keep this position for at least one to five seconds.

Forward Bend

Spread your legs out in front, keeping your hips at the same distance as your feet. Your chin should be brought to your chest so that you can stretch the ligaments between the neck and the lower portion of your skull.

Figure 30

In the same position, you can draw your elongated body to your feet by using your hands or a strap. If you're unable to reach your feet right away with your hands, you can bend your elbows and place your forearms on the ground. You can then hold your legs.

Next, you can take regular deep breaths. When you exhale, you can begin to lengthen yourself forward slowly. You may be able to maintain this posture for three minutes, or longer, if necessary.

Saddle Pose

This pose requires you to sit on your top two feet, with your shins facing away from you.

Figure 32 shows a different alternative. This is where your torso rests directly on the floor, behind your shins. You can support your torso by placing your elbows on your shoulders, your head, shoulders or any other support. You can rest your arms on the floor, with your head above your head. Keep this position for around five to ten deep breaths.

Figure 31

Figure 32

Seal Pose

Then, lay down on your stomach and face the floor. Next, create a T-shape using your arms at your sides as shown in Figure33. Also, spread your legs underneath you to create a V-shape.

Figure 33

You can raise your torso by propping on your hands. As you do this, straighten the arms. Only your torso and arms should lift off the floor. Your neck and head must remain flat. Keep the position for at least five minutes.

Square Pose

Cross your legs forward and place your left leg on the ground. Then, place the right side of your right foot on top. Keep that position for as many minutes as possible, up to six.

Figure 34

Yin Yoga Asanas may look aggressive or unfavorable, but they help stimulate certain organs. It strengthens the connective tissues, and removes blockages from meridians.

Preparing yourself for Sitting and Breathing

Yogic meditation depends on how the practitioner is seated, as well as her ability to control her breath. Yoga is a preparation for meditation.

The practitioner should seek out a tranquil environment, free from distractions and noise. It doesn't really matter where you go, so long as the environment is healthy and peaceful. You should then be relaxed. Don't get too stressed or anxious about your meditation and breathing. You can try to get rid of any negative thoughts before you even lay down on your Yoga mat.

Select the most suitable position. It is the one that you are comfortable sitting in. Choose a position you can hold throughout your meditation. In this position, you must be able to take deep and natural breaths.

It doesn't matter if your mind is occupied with distractions. But focusing on your breathing will allow you to forget about them. Be aware of how you breathe. You must be prepared to meditate.

Pranayama/Asanas are important to help you connect to your mind, spirit, and soul. Practitioners often feel stifled during yogic practices, as they cannot find the right balance between the two limbs.

They focus too much on their physical surroundings. The result is a disconnection of the mind, the body, and the spirit. This is the result of a lack of Prana (the life force which gives energy and brings peace to your mind), flowing in a complete flow.

"Breath, like life, is vital. If you breathe well, you will have a lot of it."

You will be able to live long and prosper on earth."

~ Sanskrit Proverb

The Classical

Pranayama Practices

Bandhas: Bringing them into practice

Bandha Yoga practices are the classic Yoga practices known as the energy locks or seals of the body. To perform any Bandha, you must hold the breath. This causes a slight blockage of blood circulation. Bandhas can be released which will allow energy to flow more rapidly, though it's not steady.

Why Bandhas?

Yoga students often wonder why we need to change the direction energy flows in our bodies. It is not known that the blood flow that occurs after a stoppage in blood movement can cause the body to release cells that have been long dead. This causes organs that were once home to these cells to gain a new level of strength and allows them to function properly.

Bandhas are also beneficial for the brain, since it influences Chakras as well as the Nadis responsible. You can purify your Nadis and the energy moves seamlessly from one Chakra to the next. Bandhas practice over time can help you maintain asana postures.

Bandha Types

There are four major Bandha practices that a practitioner could choose to follow. These are Mula Bandha (or Jalandhara Bandha) that can be used after inhalation. Maha Bandha (Uddiyana Bandha) and Maha Bandha (Maha Bandha) can be done after exhalation.

Mula Bandha:

Mula Bandha's practice is much easier than those of the other religions. It can be done daily. Mula actually refers to "root". To practice this Bandha the practitioner should focus on contracting between the genital and anus.

This can be done in any type of pose provided the practitioner is comfortable.

Sit down on the ground. Keep your hands on the floor and lift your torso a little. Now take a deep and sustained breath.

Press down on the floor of your pelvic region and hold it for as long as you are able.

Mula bandha is an effective way to treat sexual disorders. It gives the pelvic floor muscles more strength and firmness.

Jalandhara Bandha:

This bandha practice involves the throat and requires certain breathing techniques. Mula Bandha can take any pose that the practitioner wishes, but Jalandhara Bandha usually requires that you sit down.

Place your hands on the floor and cross your legs. Now take a deep breathe and straighten you back. Keep your eyes closed and your chin in front of your chest. You will notice a blockage in your throat.

Rest your hands on both your knees. Your shoulders should be raised and your torso should move slightly forward. Your spine should remain straight. You must maintain this position, and your breathing should be maintained.

Once you feel unable to hold your breathe, take a deep breath and exhale. You can then return to the position three or more times.

Jalandhara Bandha makes your metabolism more efficient. Also, any impurities or throat diseases can be eliminated.

Uddiyana Bandha

This is also known under the name stomach lock. It is located between the diaphragm, the pelvic floor and the stomach lock. Figure 35 shows it. This bandha redirects energy flow upward by practicing it. It is necessary to practice it in a standing or sitting position.

As you stand, take a deep inhale and hold it for a few seconds. Your hands should be resting on your knees. Now, push your torso upwards. Keep your spine straight and your shoulders lifted.

Also, make sure your legs and knees are slightly apart. Take a deep breath and hold it for as long a time as you can.

Figure 35

Uddiyana Bhag helps with constipation and indigestion. It regulates the activity of the intestine. It can also help with diabetes symptoms.

Maha Bandha

Maha bandha, also known by the names "Great Lock" (or "Great Badha"), is a constitution that all the other bandhas share. It is essential that you practice it only after you have mastered the other bandshas. These are essential to practicing the great locking. Padmasana (or a comfortable equivalent) is the pose that's most commonly required for this type of practice.

Next, take a deep inhale and exhale out of your mouth. Continue to exhale. Now, place your hands on your knees. Push your torso forwards a little.

After that, you should practice the Jalandhara Bandha. Next, move to the Uddiyana Bandha. Then stop at Mula Bandha.

You can hold your breath for as long and as you like.

Bandhas: Some precautions

You are not all meant to do bandhas. Before starting this practice, you should have learned some Pranayama breathing techniques.

Introducing Mudras into Practice

The word mudra simply means "gesture". Mudras can be described as certain postures taken by the body that alter the energy flow. They may also influence mood swings. The ancient Indians used mudras to achieve spiritual insight.

Some mudras can only be performed by the entire body. However, most are done with just the hands or the fingers. Pranayama and some meditation poses are also connected to the practice mudras.

These mudras can also be used to stimulate certain organs that control breathing and regulate Prana within the body. These mudras can also help with diseases and sickness.

Dhyana Mudra

The Dhyana or chin modra (see Figure 36) is a gesture to help connect individuals to their consciousness of self. It brings peace to mind and an overall more balanced emotional state.

Figure 36

You will need to practice chin mudra by placing your hands on your legs and opening your palms. Make a circle with your thumb and forefinger. Place the tip tip of your index finger under the thumb. Allow the rest of your fingers to spread out from these two. This mudra can be practiced in a sitting posture, with your legs crossed under each other.

The yogic representation of each of the fingers that form the circle is different for each finger. The thumb symbolizes the entire universe's consciousness. Whereas the index finger indicates the consciousness of an individual, the thumb indicates the overall consciousness. In this way, when the two forces work together, the individual becomes aware of his total being.

Garuda Mudra

This mudra, seen in Figure 37, can help the individual be more disciplined about her Yoga practice and keep it that way even when her life is hectic. The Lord Vishnu is riding the eagle.

Figure 37

Your hands should be suspended so that your palms face upwards. Now, twist your thumbs into each other. The thumbs of both your hands should meet at the base of both thumbs. Because of this, one palm is slightly below the other.

Garuda mudra is a way to increase blood flow, and also strengthen the body's organs.

Ganesha Mudra

Figure 38 is a useful mudra for relieving stress and replacing it by high spirits. It was named for Ganesha, an Indian god. He removes all obstacles from a person's way.

Figure 38

On a flat surface, you can do Padmasana or another similar pose. Or just stand. Place both your hands on your chest with your elbows bent. Turn your left palm so that your thumb faces out. With the little finger pointing at your collar bone, the thumb will shoot to the solar Plexus.

After inserting the four fingers from the right into the fingers from the left, bend each finger to face your chest. As you exhale, take deep inhalations and extend both arms keeping the eight fingers intertwined.

Dhyani Mudra

This is also known by the "meditation lock", as shown in Figure 39. It helps one achieve concentration during yogic or meditative meditation.

Figure 39

For the mudra to work, you must place the right hand on top of the left hand and rest your hands at the position of your navel. The thumbs should touch so that when they are placed together, they form a small triangle.

Dharmachakra Mudra

Dharmachakra in Sanskrit is the "wheel of dharma". It allows the individual to experience an endless flow of energy.

Figure 40

Figure 40. Place your left palm in front of your heart. Now, place your index finger and thumb on top of the ring fingers on your left hand. Your right palm should point in the opposite direction as your left.

Shiva Linga Mudra

Linga, in Sanskrit means "erect penis". This mudra aids in increasing the body's passions and heat. This mudra can also be used for fighting against severe colds. This mudra is able to be done sitting or standing.

Figure 41

As shown in Figure 41, hold both hands together, and place them on your palms. The thumb on the left should face upwards. With the index finger, and your thumb on the other hand, trace the projection of you thumb.

Vajrapradama Mudra

This is the mudra that helps build strength within the individual. Mental strength that is unwavering in self-confidence and belief of one's abilities even when there are no others.

Figure 42

As shown in Figure42, secure your fingers
with an interlace. Keep your thumbs facing
up. Continue meditation by taking slow,
steady breaths out of your nose.

Anjali Mudra

This gesture is intended to be a salutation,
particularly to the heart. This gesture helps
to alleviate stress and fears, opening up the
heart and giving the brain a calmer feeling.

You can do this in any position. As Figure 43
illustrates, place your thumb on each of
your breastbones. When you are resting
your hands on each another, let the
pressure that is being applied be as equal
and as evenly as possible. Drop your head so
that the neck of your head is parallel to your
ears. Now raise your breastbone, and then
push it into your thumbs.

Figure 43

Anjali mudra can be used to warm up for the sun salutation. It is recommended that you practice the Anjali Mudra for at least five minutes before moving on to the next sequence.

Mrigi Mudra

This is also known "deer seal". It is an important breathing technique in Pranayama. It can be used as a separate activity or combined with other breathing techniques.

Similar to Figure 44, you can also do this by fisting your right arm. Join the index and middle finger to the base. You can extend the ring and little fingers vertically with the little hand straightening and the ring finger curled towards the nail of the little.

Figure 44

Pranayama: Place your thumb on your right nostril. Press it down firmly. You will then draw in air from the left nostril. You can then block both nostrils for a moment using your thumb or ring finger. Keep the thumb in the right nostril and your ring finger in the left. The thumb should be raised and you can exhale out of the right nostril. Do the same with the left nostril. You should inhale through one nostril and keep the other closed.

Mrigi Mudra helps to alleviate headaches, and it can also help you feel more calm.

Pranayama's Four Functions

Pranayama consists of four major functions. They are: inhalation/exhalation/retention, seizure of breathe, and retention. Each of these have different yogic terms.

1. Puraka

This is the act conscious inhaling or drawing in air through your nostrils. Puraka refers to continuous breathing. Puraka practitioners are not supposed to stop inhaling.

2. Kumbhaka

This function has a relationship with inhalation. However, this function causes conscious breakage of the air and suspension of it after inhalation. This allows for storage of air in your lungs. During this time the lung is not able to move and the same goes for other parts.

3. Rechaka

Rechaka literally means "to inhale". It is the process by which the lungs release air. Similar to Puraka it is a continuous procedure.

4. Shunyaka

This is Pranayama's fourth function. It is the act of keeping air out of the lungs by closing the nostrils. We hold the breath after we exhale.

Ratios between the Exhalation, Retention, and Inhalation

6:4:6 is the regular ratio for exhalation, inhalation and retention in breathing. This means that an individual must inhale and hold the breath for at least 4 counts. After this, he should exhale after 6 counts.

Pranayama Practices

Pranayama can be practiced in many different ways. Even though they have different approaches, all of these techniques have their unique uses and benefits for Yoga.

Surya Bhedana

Surya Bhedana (or core Pranayama) is performed with the retention of breath, known as the Kumbhaka. The right nostril is the only one that can be used for breathing. As a result, all organs can be reset and are able perform their duties correctly.

Surya Bhedana is how to do it

Siddhasana, or Padmasana, can be used as a sitting position. It is important to choose a meditative pose. (We have discussed in previous chapters the best asanas suitable for Pranayama meditation). Straighten your spine. Place your hands on each knee.

Lift your right hand, and place the middle and fore finger of your right hand on your forehead. Block your left nostril and place the ring on it. Next, inhale slowly from the right nostril.

After that, you'll need to perform two bandhas: the jalandhara (or mula) bandhas. You should hold the breath as long as possible, until you are able to exhale. After that, you will need to release yourself from any bandhas. While you inhale from the left side, let the right nostril stay closed. You can continue this process for five more times. As you practice, your ability to do this will grow.

Ujjayi Pranayama

Ujjayi Pranayama also known by ocean breath, gives warmth to the skin. This breathing technique provides calmness and concentration to the mind. The lugs become completely filled with air and the throat becomes compressed. Ujjayi also has flexibility and can be done in almost all Yogic poses.

How to perform Ujjayi

You can relax by laying down in a comfortable position, your eyes closed. With your mouth slightly open, take slow deep inhale through the nostrils. Inhale and let the air flow through your throat cause the back part of your throat to contract. As air flows through the upper part of your throat, you will hear a hissing sound.

Once you have gained a grip on your throat during exhalation and inhalation, close the mouth. You will only be able to breathe through your nose. You can now contract your throat just as you did before. The sound should come from both nostrils.

Ujjayi Pranayama breathing technique says that the less air in the throat is allowed to move, the more control one has over his or her breath.

Bhastrika Pranayama

Bhastrika Pranayama can be described as a classical breathing technique, also known by the name "bellows air". It can help clear your mind and bring you to a place of understanding. Bhastrika refers to taking short deep breaths both in exhalation or inhalation. Because of this, blood movement is much faster than all other parts. The chest expands and contracts during exhalation.

How to perform Bhastrika

Make sure to find a suitable position, and keep the spine straight. Padmasana is a variant of sitting, standing, or kneeling.

Inhale and exhale forcefully, one after another through each nostril. You should ensure that your lungs have plenty of air.

Exhale hard after inhaling deeply for your first time. The hissing sound will follow.

Bhastrika refers to the use of force to breathe rapidly. Bhastrika practitioners consider it to be beneficial because it flushes out any toxins in the respiratory system. It also increases the oxygen carrying capacity of the red blood cells.

Nadi Shodhana

Nadishodana is also known by the term "alternate nostril respiration". It is the most simple, yet powerful Pranayama which allows practitioners to practice at any level of their yogic endeavours. For insomnia sufferers, it would be extremely beneficial in relieving the mind and brain from any troubled thoughts.

We already talked about Nadis, which are channels through whom Prana flows. Nadi Shodhana, which is about clearing all blocked channels caused by negative emotions (fear, stress, anxiety etc.)

How to Perform Nadi Shodhana

Sit in a comfortable and straight position. Keep your left palm resting on your thigh. Then, raise your right arm straight up and place your right thumb in line with your face.

Fold the middle and index fingers in half, letting them meet at your palm's base. Keep your thumb close to the right nostril. Next, rest the index and middle fingers near the base of the palm. Keep your thumb close to the right nostril. Deepen your left nostril by taking a slow, deep breath.

Switch to your left side nostril. Use the little finger, ring finger to block air flow through it. Keep in mind to apply gentle pressure.

You don't want your nose to be damaged. Hold your thumb against the right nostril. Take a deep breath from therein. Alternating the process for each nostril is possible.

Bhramari Prnayama

Bhramari Pranayama, also called the "hummingbee breathing technique", is a Pranayama. This Pranayama was named for its similarity with the sound a bee produces. It does wonders for the brain and forehead by calmening the nerves.

How to Perform Bhramari Pranayama

In a suitable pose, sit down. Allow your mouth to be open but keep your teeth from touching each other. Both ears can be blocked by placing the index fingers on each hand.

As your ears close, inhale deeply until the air is filled into your lungs. Release the air from the lungs by humming in your throat.

You'll feel the vibrating sound of the sound being made in your brain. For as many times you can, repeat the process.

Sheetali

Sheetali Pranayama also goes by the name "cooling Pranayama". It provides a cooling effect for the body and mind. The Sheetali way of breathing helps to regulate temperature.

How to Perform Sheetali

Once you have selected an appropriate asana, lay your palms on the knees. Your tongue should form a tube, and you can fold it from either side.

You can then take a full, deep breath. Bring your tongue back into your mouth and close it.

Drop your neck to perform Jalandhara Bandha. You should hold the pose for as long time as you can. After you reach the point of yielding, exhale deeply into your nose.

Murcha Pranayama

First, Murcha Pranayama can be recommended to those who are already able to do other Pranayama methods. It is important that the person maintain a certain posture until they feel the need to pass out.

It is possible to feel a long-lasting sustenance of your breath as it enters the nostrils. There is also a locking of your chin near the thyroid gland. People who are successful in practicing Murchapranayama often feel joy and other positive emotions.

How to do Murccha Pranayama

Find an asana that suits you. You can inhale and exhale using both your nostrils. Continue inhaling for five more counts.

Your head should be in the direction of your chest and chin. You should hold this position for five seconds. After five seconds, let the breath leave your nostrils.

Plavini Pranayama

Plavini literally means "to flot". Plavini is an example of someone who is drinking air, instead of water. There is an increase in stomach size. Plavini Pranayama practitioners are able to work for hours on end without needing to eat.

The atmosphere has enough energy to allow for breathing.

It is described in verse 70 the second chapter Hatha Yoga Pradipika.

"Due to the abundance of air drawn in, the Yogi is able to float easily in deep waters. It's like a lotus leaf."

How to Perform Plavini

You can sit comfortably in an asana and draw your breath through both nostrils. The Jalahandhra bhajan helps you to retain your breath.

This will allow for more circulation to the stomach, intestines and lungs. Once your stomach is bloated, exhale deeply through each nostril.

Kapalabhati Pranayama

Kapalabhati Pranayama focuses on the practice of inhaling deeply and short exhaled, but not too deep. It is a cleansing agent for the respiratory system and lungs. You can also strengthen your abdominal muscles by continuing to practice.

How to Perform Kapalabhati Pranayama

As always, maintain a comfortable position by bending your spine and keeping your abdomen open. Place your hands down on your knees with your palms facing downwards.

As an alternative, focus on the lower stomach by placing your two hands on it. Now take a deep inhale through both nostrils. You can then compress your lower stomach to let the air out.

Once you've released your body from compression, exhalation will become voluntary. This allows you to focus your exhalation on the task at hand.

Anulom Olom Pranayama

Anulom Vilom a technique for alternate nostril breath that can be practiced with no need to hold your breath.

How to Perform Anulom Vilom

You can find a comfortable asana to sit in, most preferably the Padmasana. Block your right nostril with your thumb, and then inhale through you left nostril. Continue to inhale till the lugs become full.

After that, you can release your thumb. Now inhale through the right side of your nose.

Switch the procedure to inhale from your right nostril while exhaling through the left. This is the longest you can keep going.

It is important to realize that all of these breathing techniques can be used to clear the mind. Meditation is impossible if you don't have a clear mind.

Feelings change like clouds in a windy day.

My anchor is mindful breathing.

Thich Nhat Hanh

Your Pranayama Practice

Precautions & Contraindications

Pranayama practice is not without its limitations. These are signs that make Pranayama not recommended for certain people. These are just a few of the warning signs and contraindications you should know.

Pranayama: Some precautions

1. Pranayama is not recommended for anyone with serious medical conditions. Certain conditions, such as heart disease

or asthma, might prevent you from pranayama.

2. Pranayama is the eight limbs that make up Yoga practice. Pranayamas are best started once you have mastered certain postures (asana). Pranayama regulates Prana's movement within the body. Asanas, which help to remove closures in Nadis responsible for this Prana, are essential.

3. Pranayama can be done after you've eaten. Between meals and Pranayama, there should be a reasonable time gap. A minimum of three hours should be allowed between activities, especially if you've just eaten a substantial meal.

4. Pranayama requires that you breathe through the nose. You should not try to retain your breath when you first start practicing Pranayama. You should only do

this under the guidance of a Yoga instructor.

5. Pranayama can be difficult for those who feel tired and uncomfortable. It is important to stop Pranayama immediately in order to rest and relax. You can warm up by taking long, deep breathes before returning to Pranayama.

6. Pranayama should always be done in an open area. Inadequate ventilation can cause shortness or even death.

Pranayama Contraindications

Here are some side effects that Pranayama could cause.

1. Dizziness

2. Headache

3. Indigestion

4. Blurred vision

5. Nauseating effects

Preparing Your Environment

Spaces for Practice and Education

Pranayama can be practiced in a variety of ways. The ideal space to practice Pranayama in is one that is clean and well ventilated. It should also be quiet, as a calm environment is key to a peaceful mind.

Also, you can prepare for your practice by keeping a piece of interest in your space. It will act as an unconsciously connected object to your mind while you breathe. You can think of it as a motivation to perform.

Customizing Your Personal Practice

Pranayama (and Yoga) should always be begun with an instructor, or in a Yoga class. But it is also important that you establish a practice schedule. You will find your Prana becomes more manageable if you have one that is familiar to your body.

Where?

This idea has been covered before. Pranayama practice is best done in a well-ventilated space. It is best to choose a place in your house that is not too comfortable. If you are tempted to lay down and practice, you should leave the bedroom. You could also look at another space in the house that has a comfortable and flat floor.

Setting your practice intentions

For this reason, it is important to consider the following:

1. Pranayama can be practiced anywhere in your house.

2. What timeframe do you prefer for your sessions to take place?

3. How many hours do you want to practice in a session?

4. What do YOU want your practice area to look like

Scheduling Practice time

Pranayama works best in the early mornings, when there is less tension and the sun still has not yet risen in the sky. You can practice pranayama at other times throughout the day.

How long does it take?

Pranayama daily can be very helpful. Every day, you can practice Pranayama for around fifteen minutes. Pranayama can be difficult to master. It requires patience.

Build Your Practice Space

You can have the following items in your practice:

* a Yoga mat

* Blankets

* Blocks

* Belts or elastic ropes

* any object to invoke a spiritual atmosphere, such as an adornment, ritual, and/or object.

Using A Pranayama Journal

Pranayama can be practiced by keeping journals that cover breathing and Pranayama. They are often filled with tips and guidelines on breathing. There are other topics that may not be covered in this book but can be found in magazines or publications that focus on Pranayama. Keep a journal of your Yoga practice to aid you in your yogic pursuits.